Heels vs. Ties

Living With Your #1 Threat

Cynthia Cunningham

By: Dr. Nitza I Alvarez

Because we love what you do for our kids we want to share this gift of life.

Heart Disease claim the lives of thousand women even year.

Refuse To Be Just Another Statistic!

1

Heels vs. Ties is not intended as a substitute for medical advice. Consult your own doctor before implementing any of the recommendations that the author offers in this book.

What is intended from this book is to empower you to take care of your health and become your own advocate. It's to stop you from becoming a statistic and change the sad truth that heart disease is the #1 killer of women.

Take control of your health.

#PreventTheStent

Published by: RI-AL Consulting

Edited by: Leesa Klich

Written by: Dr. Nitza I Alvarez

Cover Design by: Red Apples Media

Cover Photo by: RI-AL Consulting

ISBN-13: 978-0692191576
ISBN-10: 0692191577

First edition March 2019

Social Media

www.tc-heart.com

www.heelsvsties.com

https://www.facebook.com/tricountyheartinstitute

@TriCountyHeart

For educational videos visit:

https://www.youtube.com/channel/UCPKA1uBL_Ih
VGTwmw_S1YEg

Be your own advocate

Don't stop until you get an answer.

Dedication

- For those who died for not recognizing their symptoms on time.
- For those women who learn about their risk too late.
- For the mothers that worry about others and place themselves last.
- To the family and friends whom I have lost.
- To women everywhere that stay silent, living with their #1 life threat: **Heart Disease.**

Prevention is the most important intervention.

#PreventTheStent

Did you know?

✓ Heart disease, also known as cardiovascular disease, is the leading cause of death in the United States, causing more than 420,000 deaths among women every year.

✓ 50,000 more women than men die of heart disease every year.

✓ More women than men die because women tend to be underdiagnosed and undertreated for heart disease symptoms.

✓ Over eight million American women live with heart disease.

✓ Each year more women die from heart disease than all cancers combined.

✓ For every woman that dies from breast cancer there are six that die from heart disease.

Table of Contents

Introduction

Medical research has historically neglected the health needs of women, apart from reproductive concerns. This is what we like to call the "Bikini Approach" or the "Gender Gap."

Just a couple of decades ago heart disease was considered strictly a man's disease and, even though we have come a long way, doctors are still practicing medicine based on studies performed in white middle-aged men.

This is why I named the book *Heels vs. Ties*. Today in our society Heels have an unquestionably feminine association, while Ties are a must-have clothing accessory for men. Contrasting these two objects is done intentionally to emphasize that we are different, that there are clear differences in risks, symptoms, presentation, diagnosis, and treatment of heart disease in women.

This book is intended to promote awareness of the increased risk that we as women have of dying from a medical condition that is preventable.

Before we begin, let me share with you a story about one of the patients under my care to help illustrate how symptoms of heart disease can show up in unexpected ways. Sometimes these seemingly unrelated symptoms can be improved when you address the heart.

Mrs. N. was a 63-year-old woman that had difficulty breathing. Her major complaint was that she couldn't complete simple tasks at home like sweeping the floors, dusting, and making her bed without having to stop because she couldn't breathe.

At the beginning, her shortness of breath was related to physical activity, however she noticed this changed about three months earlier. Mrs. N. saw a lung doctor who prescribed inhalers for her newly diagnosed lung condition known as COPD (chronic obstructive pulmonary disease). After three months with her inhalers she had not noticed any improvement in her symptoms.

On our first visit she told me that she felt more fatigued than usual for the past few months, and she also experienced episodes of "achy" pain in her upper back between her shoulder blades from time-to-time. She had seen a chiropractor, however the last few sessions had not been effective in alleviating her discomfort. On her physical exam she had high blood pressure and no other significant findings were noted. Her lab tests revealed high cholesterol and mildly elevated blood sugar levels. Based on her symptoms, I suggested a test that would look for blockages in the blood vessels of the heart, as this would show an increased risk for a heart attack. She disagreed and went back to see her chiropractor one more time.

Her symptoms worsened and she came back to see me. This time I had her tested. Her test results suggested that she had some injury to her heart muscle and needed more tests to confirm. Additional testing done found that she had severe narrowing or blockages in two of the major arteries of her heart.

After receiving proper treatment to reduce the blocked arteries, including intervention and medical therapy, her back pain, shortness of breath, fatigue all improved, and she recovered her lifestyle.

Never ignore your symptoms

The heart is a vital organ, I like to call it THE organ that keep us alive.

What is Heart Disease?

When we think of heart disease, we often picture a man grabbing his chest in pain from a heart attack. But there's a lot more going on in the body for years (even decades) beforehand that led up to that point.

Let's start with the definition. Heart disease is also known as cardiovascular disease. The *cardio* refers to the heart itself and *vascular* is for vessels like arteries and veins that run throughout the whole body. So, heart (or cardiovascular) *disease* refers to medical conditions that affect the heart and vessels. There are many different medical conditions including:

- Coronary Artery Disease (CAD): A disease of the vessels that supply blood to your heart muscle (yes, your heart needs its own arteries). This is a long-term condition that increases your risk for, and can eventually lead to, a heart attack.

- Heart Attack: When your heart gets injured because it did not receive appropriate blood flow through the coronary arteries that supply nutrients and oxygen to the heart muscle itself.

This is also known as *myocardial infarction*, or *MI*, and is often the result of many years living with risk factors that you might not even know, such as high cholesterol, hypertension, diabetes, smoking, poor eating habits, and lack of exercise.

- Peripheral Vascular Disease (PVD): A disease of the arteries that supply the rest of your body, beyond your heart. Also known as Peripheral Arterial Disease (PAD).

- Heart Failure (HF): A condition in which the heart doesn't pump blood effectively. Either because it is weak or it cannot fill properly.

- Arrhythmia: Irregular heartbeat. A variation of the normal beat of the heart.

Measure your risk of coronary artery disease (CAD)

You're probably wondering if you are at risk for heart disease and what you can do about it.

Let's start by taking a look at your risk factors with this simple quiz. After that, read on to learn more about how you, as a woman, can reduce your risk and #PreventTheStent.

Answer the ten quick yes or no questions below giving yourself one point every time your answer is *yes*.

1.Have you reached menopause? In other words, have you not had a menstrual period for 12 consecutive months? Y

2.Are you fifty-five-years old or older? Y

3.Did one of your parents or siblings have a heart attack or sudden cardiac death before the age of 55 (males) or 65 (females)? N

4.Have you smoked cigarettes in the past 10 years? N

5.Is your blood pressure 130/80 or higher, or do you take medications for high blood pressure? __N__

6.Does at least one of these apply to you:

- Is your total cholesterol 200 mg/dL or higher?
- Is your LDL 160 mg/dL or higher?
- Are your triglycerides 150 ml/dL or higher?
- Do you take medications for any of these? __1__

7.Do you have diabetes or high blood sugars? __1__

8. Are you overweight or obese? __Y__

Calculate your Body Mass Index

BMI = 703 x (weight (lb)/ height (in)2)

Overweight: BMI 25-29.9

Obesity: BMI 30+

9.Are you physically active for less than 30 consecutive minutes per day? __Y__

10.Do you worry excessively, and/or suffer from insomnia, headaches, stomach problems, or fatigue? __Y__

Add the total points.

My score is __5-1__

If your score is at least two, you have a moderate risk for heart attack. If your score is five or higher, you have a high risk for heart attack.

This quiz is based on the Framingham Risk Score: the accepted tool to measure risk of heart disease. It has new risks added to better understand the risks women have of developing CAD.

Note that when it comes to age, women have a higher risk of developing heart disease after the age of fifty-five; but this does not mean that you cannot have heart disease at younger age.

We are going to talk about these dangers right after we briefly go over coronary artery disease, cholesterol, and heart attacks.

If you are not experiencing any symptom but you know you are at risk for heart disease, you should be evaluated or examine. Prevention is the most important intervention.

#PreventTheStent

Coronary Artery Disease

The heart is a vital organ, I like to call it *the* organ that keeps us alive; however, as with every other part of our body, it needs to be nourished. The nutrients and oxygen it needs to be healthy are carried in the blood that reaches the heart muscle through the coronary arteries.

Coronary artery disease (CAD) is the type of heart disease that affects the arteries supplying the heart muscle itself. It is the most common form of heart disease. But sadly, according to a statement released by the American Heart Association (AHA) in January of 2016, this condition is underdiagnosed, undertreated, and under-researched in women. The conclusion of this statement is sad, but for the first time in the ninety-three-year history of the AHA, the organization decided to finally issue an official statement about women and heart attack.

Why the differences between men and women?

Medical research has historically neglected the health needs of women, apart from reproductive concerns. This is what we like to call the

"Bikini Approach" or the "Gender Gap."

Is it an incomplete understanding of the disease?

Is it that women have more risk factors?

Perhaps it is that CAD in women is a different disease altogether?

What causes CAD?

CAD is known to be caused by atherosclerosis (a buildup of plaque inside the walls of the arteries). This accumulation narrows the vessels that supply blood and oxygen to the heart.

In women, CAD might happen even *without* severe plaque buildup. Women are more likely to have *unusual* ways of developing CAD. Compared to men, women with heart attacks usually have less plaque in their arteries to explain the cause of the obstruction of blood flow to the heart muscle.

When plaques form on the walls of the arteries it also causes inflammation. Plaque formation is encouraged in several ways:

Plaque: *Mix of cholesterol, calcium, and scar tissue.*

Inflammation: *When the body's immune system reacts to infections, wounds or tissue damage. When it occurs for a long time it can eventually lead to several diseases or conditions.*

- Increased concentrations of *bad* cholesterol (LDL: low-density lipoprotein) circulating in your blood (see definition for lipoprotein at the end of this section).

- Decreased concentrations of *good* cholesterol (HDL: high-density lipoprotein) in your blood. These particles are heart healthy because they remove bad cholesterol from your circulation.

- High blood pressure may enhance the penetration of LDL into the arterial walls, promoting injury. This leads to your blood vessels becoming stiffer and weaker over time.

- Damage to the interior part of your arteries promoted by toxins such as nicotine.

- High blood sugar affects the proper handling of triglycerides resulting in high levels in your blood. It also increases the oxidation of the LDL making it more harmful. An example of oxidation is rusting of metals. You don't want your LDL to get too oxidized. (We'll talk about blood sugar and diabetes later in the book.)

Over time the plaque grows and hardens in your arteries, causing them to become narrower. A simple way to visualize this concept is with the analogy of a clogged water hose. Despite a good flow of water coming from the faucet, the water flow that you see coming out into your garden is limited because of the clog. If the clog is not taken care of, the plants can end up dying.

> **Lipoprotein:** *A group of proteins capable of mixing with water or blood that combine with fat to transport it through your bloodstream. LDL is low-density lipoprotein (sometimes called bad cholesterol) and HDL is high-density lipoprotein (sometimes called good cholesterol). See the next chapter on cholesterol for more information.*
>
> **Triglycerides** *(TGs): The most common type of fat in your body. When your blood level of TGs are too high, this is a risk for heart disease.*

What is Cholesterol?

Is cholesterol all bad? Despite the bad reputation that cholesterol might have, human beings cannot live without it. Cholesterol does some very important things in the body:

- It's needed for the production of membranes in every cell of your body.

- It's a critical ingredient to make sex hormones, including estrogen.

- We need cholesterol to produce vitamin D which is essential for the absorption of calcium.

- It's used to make bile to absorb fat from our meals.

Our body is capable of producing the cholesterol that we need to help our bodies function properly. Normally, the more cholesterol we get from our food, the less we produce on our own. When we eat too much saturated fat from our diets (i.e., from meat and dairy), the excess gets stored in the liver. The body has a wonderful mechanism to notice when the liver has stored enough, and it reduces the amount of cholesterol it produces.

However, if you are consuming excess of it your levels will remain elevated in your blood.

When there is more cholesterol circulating in your body, this increases the deposit of cholesterol into artery walls and produces plaque in our vessels, contributing to atherosclerosis.

Where do LDL and HDL come from?

Cholesterol is basically fat, and fat cannot dissolve in water, nor in blood; therefore, in order to travel through the bloodstream, fat must be carried as a complex molecule called a *lipoprotein*. Lipoproteins are produced in many parts of the body. They are like little goblets of fat that transport cholesterol through your bloodstream. Those particles, called lipoproteins, contain two kinds of fat which are important sources of energy: cholesterol and triglycerides. These ingredients are combined with proteins which allows the fat to successfully dissolve in the blood.

Whether our body gets the cholesterol from the food we eat, or produces it itself, the cholesterol must be converted or broken down into a form that can be used by the body. When we eat fat, there are miniature fat molecules that are formed which get absorbed into the bloodstream. In the process, these get broken down further and are converted into triglycerides.

Most of the triglycerides will deposit in fatty tissue throughout your body, but some are broken up when they get delivered to your liver. What is left of that triglyceride that did not reach the liver is allowed to remain in the bloodstream. After a series of complicated steps, the liver will repackage the smaller particles of fat. These particles are called LDL (low-density lipoprotein) and HDL (high-density lipoprotein).

Effects of LDL

LDL is the major carrier of cholesterol in our body and it has been identified as the major culprit for plaque formation. It delivers the cholesterol to the cells of the body where it's taken in and is used to repair the cell.

When the cells have enough cholesterol to do their repair work, they slowdown in taking in any more cholesterol from the blood, so it stays there. It is these high levels of cholesterol in your bloodstream that can actually cause the plaque formation.

Your doctor can do a blood test called a *lipid profile* to verify your LDL number. This will give her or him an idea if you have too much of it, and can also measure the

circulating particles known as LDLp (pretty cool, ah?).
The size of the particles matter as some of them are more
prone to get stuck in the walls of the vessels and cause
plaques and atherosclerosis

Effects of HDL

What about your HDL? HDL is known as the *superman* of
the cholesterols. Its principal job is to carry the unused
cholesterol in the blood and bring it back to the liver to
be excreted as bile. The bile empties into the intestine,
flushing excess cholesterol out of the body in your stool.

Any excess cholesterol still in your blood is considered a
high risk for heart disease, with the exception of HDL.

> You want your cholesterol report to have
>
> "Low LDL, High HDL."

Links between cholesterol and heart disease

Based on research of the links between high cholesterol
and heart disease, the American Heart Association (AHA)
recommends total cholesterol levels of 200 mg/dL or less.
If your numbers are higher than this, you will want to
know what your LDL, triglycerides, and HDL are.

We have learned that, for women:

- Total cholesterol is an important risk factor for the related condition, stroke.

- Low levels of HDL cholesterol and/or high levels of triglycerides are dangerous and strong predictors of heart disease.

When to get your cholesterol checked

Cholesterol has been circulating in our bodies since we were born, therefore I believe that every woman should have a complete lipid profile taken by their thirtieth birthday and definitely before menopause.

If your results are abnormal you will need close monitoring and changes to your lifestyle including more physical activity, a heart-healthy diet, and if needed, medications. If you have a parent, sibling, or grandparent with high blood lipids, you should have a lipid profile test done at the age of 18. If you are a woman that plans to start or continue on an oral contraceptive pill you should have your lipids monitored at least annually. Sometimes all you'll need is to make some lifestyle changes including diet and exercise. If that's not enough, your doctor will design the treatment with you.

Am I in danger?

Now, let's go through some of the items from the quiz to understand the roles they play in your risk of heart disease.

What roles do age and menopause play in heart disease risk?

Cardiovascular risk factors in women increase in the menopausal years. We don't know exactly whether this increased risk is related to aging, hormonal changes, or both. Hormones like estrogen that are present prior to menopause may protect against CAD (coronary artery disease) and may explain the approximately 10 year later onset of CAD in women compared to men. The incidence of heart attack in women with normal estrogen levels is very low (1-7 percent per 100,000). It is 3-5 times lower than in men.

However, this favorable association decreases in older women (sixty-five years of age and older). Several large research studies have shown that premature menopause (i.e., before the age of fifty-three) increases the risk of CAD, particularly in women who smoke. Estrogen seems to prevent plaque formation and hardening of the plaque. The decline in estrogen production leads to various, usually annoying symptoms (like hot flashes), obesity, atrophy of your genitalia, memory problems, and eventually to an increased risk of developing diseases like osteoporosis and heart disease, among others. The heart is one of the organs significantly affected by menopause. The estrogen deficiency results in increased thickening of your heart muscle, heart failure, and changes in how your body manages cholesterol causing elevation of your *bad* cholesterol (LDL) and triglycerides.

> **Clot:** *When some of the blood component clump together, as in a scab that forms when you cut your skin.*

Menopause also leads to increased levels of substances that promote dangerous clot formation inside your blood vessels. The combination of both plaque and clot formation increases the risk of ruptured plaques that can block the flow of blood through the vessel. This blockage can lead to a heart attack. The high concentration of certain factors in the blood that promote clotting is believed to be associated with heart disease.

Your age and hormones also influence a number of other, not so obvious, risk factors for heart disease.

Is my age giving me a belly?

You may have noticed your belly getting larger. As women age, especially after menopause, the proportion of body fat in the midsection increases.

In menopausal women this is the result of the decline of production of estrogen and the activation of a substance that increases the breakdown of cholesterol (known as *lipoprotein lipase*) in your abdomen. Both lead to the accumulation of fat in the abdominal region. The consequence of this process is that abdominal fat increases the risk for heart disease and death.

High levels of abdominal fat includes fat you can't see that is around your internal organs. This deeper fat is known as *visceral adipose tissue*. When this is present there is an increase in inflammation which "rusts" the LDL particles making them more damaging. To make matters worse the adipose tissue prevents other compounds that help reduce the oxidation of those "rusted" particles and disposes of them to prevent damage to the lining of the vessels and more plaque from forming.

Does age influence my blood sugar levels?

Women with low estrogen levels or high levels of male hormones (e.g., with polycystic ovarian syndrome: PCOS) have an increased risk of developing high blood sugar or diabetes in the future. You'll remember from the quiz that diabetes or high blood sugar is one of the major risk factors for heart disease.

How does age affect my blood pressure?

High blood pressure is an important risk factor for heart disease and the related condition, stroke. Although the systolic blood pressure (the top number of your blood pressure reading) is higher in men compared to women under forty-years old, for people over sixty-years old the systolic blood pressure is higher in women. The diastolic blood pressure (the bottom number) gradually increases in a similar pattern in both genders as they age. A woman's blood pressure increases significantly between the first and fifth year after the onset of menopause.

> **Stroke:** *A condition that happens when your brain doesn't get enough oxygenated blood.*

Can I turn back the clock using hormones?

After all this talk about the protective effects that estrogen has on our hearts, you may be wondering about hormonal therapy. Menopausal hormone therapy has been widely used to try to restore the hormonal environment to the premenopausal state. This is only to treat menopausal symptoms, but will they help to "turn back the clock" regarding heart disease risk? Recent research has not shown that hormone therapy offers protection from heart attacks, and in fact, they have shown potential harm in older women. There are still many unanswered questions regarding the benefits and risks of menopausal hormonal treatment, specifically relating to heart disease in women. There are several factors to consider when it comes to whether hormonal therapy is right for you. These include: type of hormone, timing, how much to take (dosage), how to take it, and how long to take it for.

Taking hormone replacement therapy to prevent heart disease is controversial. There are dozens of studies designed to evaluate heart attacks and other health consequences in women receiving hormone replacement therapy, however, the recommendations continue to be *not* to use them for prevention of heart disease. Taking hormonal pills has been linked to increased risk of heart attacks, breast cancer, and clot formation, among other problems. Interestingly, a recent study in a large group of post-menopausal women showed that women who took hormone replacement therapy had a lower coronary calcium score which indicates a decreased risk for heart disease. I believe that all women would benefit from a better understanding of the associations between reproductive hormones, cardiovascular health, and hormone therapy risk, and get guidance regarding appropriate actions to take to protect their heart health. Together we can advocate for more research to understand this important aspect of our health.

I'm young with no family history of heart disease why should I worry?

Nobody is exempt from heart disease. For example, your heart disease can be there from birth such as irregular heartbeats (arrhythmias) or abnormalities in the heart structure itself. Although they might be diagnosed during your childhood they may not be found until pregnancy, or even later.

Heart disease and pregnancy

Heart disease associated with pregnancy is common. Conditions such as gestational diabetes (a form of diabetes that appears during pregnancy) and/or high blood pressure that commonly occur during pregnancy, significantly increase the risk of a heart attack later in life. One in five women in the United States has a form of these conditions during at least one pregnancy. With more professional women waiting to start their family later in life, and with the increased incidence of obesity and diabetes, the number of women at risk for these pregnancy complications continues to rise. Unfortunately, most women are unaware of these disorders. But what is more unthinkable is that many healthcare providers are unaware that these disorders during pregnancy significantly increase the risk of heart attacks later in life.

Have you been asked by your doctor if you've had any of these conditions? If you have had any of them please know that your risk for any heart condition is higher. Take control by seeing a doctor that listens to you and takes you seriously.

Expectant mothers

Pregnancy is a time of dramatic changes in a woman's body and in many respects mimics an early stress test.

Accommodations for the growing fetus increases the size and number of blood vessels; creates changes in the amount of blood, heart size, and pumping capacity; and increases the vulnerability of your arteries to damage.

Several heart problems commonly affect pregnant women including the rupture of some of the blood vessels and a reduction in the heart's ability to properly pump blood in the late stages of pregnancy or shortly after delivery.

Often, these conditions occur suddenly and tend to be life-threatening for both mother and child. Doctors often do tests or prescribe therapies on these two vulnerable patients with little or no scientific evidence to support their decisions. We have a critical knowledge gap regarding optimal care for the mother and the baby when heart disease complicates pregnancy. This is because pregnant women and women of reproductive age are almost always excluded from clinical research.

Stress Test: An exercise stress test that is one of the most commonly used tests to reveal hidden problems in the heart making your heart work harder. It is similar to what a mechanic does when checking your car

Compared to men, women with heart attacks usually have less plaque in their arteries to explain the cause of the obstruction of blood flow to the heart muscle.

High blood pressure (the silent killer)

High blood pressure (hypertension) is also known as the *silent killer* because it has no symptoms and often goes undiagnosed, yet is a huge contributor to heart disease deaths. In 2013 more than 360,000 American deaths were from high blood pressure.

Hypertension is very common in industrialized nations with more than twenty percent of the general population having it, and many don't even know it. High blood pressure increases greatly with age, affecting only 5.9 percent of women aged eighteen to forty-four, but rising to 39.1 percent of women aged forty-five to sixty-four. For women aged sixty-five and older, nearly three in four (74.4 percent) have high blood pressure.

High blood pressure also varies by race and ethnicity. A 2009-2010 study showed that over 40 percent of African-American women had hypertension, compared to about 25 percent of Caucasian and Hispanic women. However, 44.8 percent of women studied with uncontrolled hypertension reported that they had never received a diagnosis from a doctor.

High blood pressure increases your risk for dangerous health conditions such as:

- First heart attack: About seven out of every ten people who experience their first heart attack have high blood pressure.

- Heart failure (long-term): About seven of every ten people with chronic heart failure have high blood pressure.

- Other related conditions like stroke and kidney disease (gradual loss of kidney function where the kidneys fail to filter waste products from the blood properly).

When your blood pressure is high, your blood vessels lose elasticity and become stiffer and less flexible, leading to heart disease. This results in damage to the vessels. How this injury happens is not very well understood.

This injury causes plaque formation in specific areas of the blood vessels, not throughout their whole length. The majority of the plaque buildup appears to happen around areas where the artery twists or branches. This is believed to occur as a reaction to unstable blood flow due to blood pressure. If the blood flow is altered there is an increase in the pulsing of the blood flow and the pressure is increased. This pressure between circulating blood and the lining of the vessel finally results in the lining becoming disrupted (the injury) and plaque starting to build up.

Another mechanism through which high blood pressure may be involved in heart attacks is through rupture of the plaque. When a plaque builds up inside a vessel, and that vessel has high pressure inside it, pieces of that plaque can break off, or rupture. The rupture of the plaque causes the blood inside that vessel to clot because the body treats this rupture like an injury. This is similar to the clot (scab) that forms when you cut your skin. Because this is happening inside a small vessel, the clot grows and blocks the flow of blood through that vessel. This can result in a heart attack.

When your blood pressure is high, your heart works harder, causing it more stress. In addition, high blood pressure will initially make your heart muscle get thicker as any muscle will do when it is working against high resistance. Take a look at somebody that lifts heavy weights regularly, their muscles are bigger. However, if the high blood pressure is not controlled, the heart will eventually get weak through remodeling of the muscle that grows without appropriate blood flowing to that area.

Through this process you might experience symptoms of heart failure, which I will discuss in another chapter.

Remodeling: Many different diseases, including hypertension, can alter the performance of the heart. With high blood pressure, in order for the heart to continue supplying nutrients and oxygen throughout the body, the heart cells change their shape and arrangement to compensate. This and other adaptations together will result in myocardial remodeling.

What makes my blood pressure increase?

There are several factors that can increase your blood pressure. They are:

- Not doing at least 30 minutes of physical activity per day.
- Having excess weight or obesity.
- Having atherosclerosis (plaque and stiffening of the arteries).
- Feeling a lot of stress.
- Eating too much salt (if you are salt sensitive, even a small amount can significantly affect your blood pressure).

When your doctor talks about salt, this goes beyond your salt shaker. Processed food, sauces, hot dogs, hamburgers, pre-packaged meals, canned food, mustard, ketchup, and many others, are loaded with salt.

What can I do about high blood pressure?

There are a few things you can do for high blood pressure:

- Follow a heart-healthy diet.
- Limit salt intake.
- Meditate to reduce stress.
- Take your medications as suggested by your doctor.
- Be physically active.

The recommendation of the American Heart Association (AHA) is to do aerobic exercise at least 2.5 hours per week. 30 minutes of moderate-intensity activity five days per week. Good examples of aerobic exercises are: walking, jogging, swimming, or biking. For those 30 minutes, 15 minutes should be continuous aerobic exercise. Less than this in a session is better than nothing, but will not be as effective in reducing your risk of heart disease.

New studies show that this time can be divided in a few days if you are too busy.

There is nothing atypical about women's heart attack symptoms other than they are not the symptoms that are typically experienced by men.

Sweet heart - Elevated sugar

The word diabetes was first recorded in 1425, the Greek *mellitus*, "like honey," was added, to reflect the sweet smell and taste of the patient's urine.

Diabetes is a condition where there are high sugar levels in your blood. This results from the body's inability to use blood sugar for energy.

There are two types of diabetes, both involving the hormone insulin. Insulin is key for managing blood sugar because it helps the sugar get out of your blood and into the cells where it can be used for energy.

In type 1 diabetes, the body no longer makes insulin and therefore blood sugar cannot leave the blood and enter the cells to be used for energy.

In type 2 diabetes, either the body can no longer make enough insulin, or the body is unable to use insulin correctly. This happens in both sexes, however, estrogen levels influence glucose metabolism.

One of the most severe complications of diabetes is the early onset of atherosclerosis. Women with diabetes seem to have a higher risk of developing heart disease than men with diabetes. Having diabetes nearly doubles your chance of having a heart attack.

Diabetes promotes plaque formation in many ways. First of all, high blood sugar levels damage the lining of the vessels, initiating plaque buildup. This then starts a series of events that promote formation and growth of the plaque.

Diabetes affects all the blood vessels in the body, large and small. When the small vessels are affected you are prone to develop problems in areas of the body with small vessels which can lead to blindness, kidney failure, and nerve damage. However, when the large vessels are involved, the complications include heart attack and stroke. The amount of damage is related to how long and how severe the high blood sugar problems are.

If you have diabetes, your major goal should be to control your blood sugar levels by following your doctor's instructions regarding your medications. It is also very important to focus on weight loss and diet.

If your doctor has mentioned that you have prediabetes, you still have time to reduce your risk of developing diabetes. As the American Diabetes Association (ADA) states, you will not automatically develop type 2 diabetes if you have prediabetes. For some people with prediabetes, early treatment can actually return blood sugar levels to normal. Make sure that you are tested for diabetes if you:

- Are forty-five-years old or older.

- Are forty-years old or older if you are overweight or obese (and repeat testing every three years if results are normal).

- Are an American Indian, Alaskan Native, Asian American, Hispanic or Latino, or a Native Hawaiian or Pacific Islander.

- Have a personal history of gestational diabetes or polycystic ovarian syndrome.

Having diabetes nearly doubles your chance of having a heart attack.

Why weight loss and diet are so important

Here's why focusing on weight loss and diet is so important and why you should watch what you eat. The main source of fuel for our body is sugar. Your body uses both naturally-occurring sugar from fruits and vegetables, as well as sugar added to ultra-processed food. Ultra-processed foods include everything that has been milled, canned, cooked, frozen, or dehydrated; however, these on their own do not necessarily make them bad. What makes them bad is the *number* of changes the ingredients go through as food manufacturers improve flavor, color, and shelf life. For example, milling of grains will remove the bran and the germ which contain most of the healthy fiber, protein, vitamins, and minerals; however, there has been no significant modification of the ingredients. Another example is the addition of sugar or salt to food which makes it less healthy. Canned foods, sugar coated dried fruits, soda, sugary or savory packaged snack foods, packaged breads and pastries, breaded chicken nuggets and fish, and instant noodle soups are all examples of ultra-processed foods. Look for other additives and trans fats listed in the Nutrition Facts table (See Appendix I for a table of the most common food additives). If you can eat whole foods the way nature provides them, this is better. However, some ultra-processed foods might offer valuable nutrients.

The moral of the story is: Read the labels.

If you have a high caloric intake the excess calories will be store for the future--as fat (See Appendix III for a table of the calorie needs for women). This is why your cholesterol can remain elevated even when you have been avoiding fat intake in your diet--you might be getting excess calories from protein or carbohydrates. Ultra-processed food is often high in calories with minimal nutrients, and increases inflammation which increases your risk for plaque formation.

Research shows that you can lower your risk for type 2 diabetes by 58 percent by:

- Losing seven percent of your body weight (or 15 pounds if you weigh 200 pounds). Don't worry if you can't get to your ideal body weight. Losing even 10 pounds can make a huge difference!
- Being moderately physically active (such as brisk walking) 30 minutes per day, five days per week.

> Abdominal fat increases the risk for
> heart disease and death.

Cigarettes

According to the latest statistics from the Centers for Disease Control and Prevention (CDCP), nearly 14 of every 100 adult women (13.5 percent) smoke. Smoking has been associated with increased risk for heart disease.

I'm pretty sure that if you smoke you know that you are

> Despite the fact that almost everyone associates cigarettes with lung disease, smoking is the cause of about 30 percent of heart disease.

not doing your body any good. Despite the relaxing feeling that nicotine might give you as it alters the balance of chemicals in your brain, the nicotine in cigarettes increases your blood pressure and your resting heart rate (pulse) adding more stress to your heart. Smoking also makes your blood stickier, increasing the chance of blood clot formation inside the blood vessels, and lowers your oxygen levels depriving your heart of it. Through these and other mechanisms, smoking increases the plaque formation in your arteries.

If you are an active smoker, if you used to smoke less than 10 years ago, or if you are exposed to second-hand smoke, then you have an additional risk factor for heart disease. Women who smoke have a 25 percent higher risk of developing heart disease compared to men who smoke. Take action and eliminate the cigarettes from your life!

I understand that when it comes to quitting smoking it is easier said than done. Many times, women use cigarettes as a way of coping with stress and frustration. As a doctor to many women that have been in the same position that you might be in at this moment, I understand that it is not an easy task. The rush and the "feel good" reasons make it hard to quit, however the good news is that there are many ways to get help quitting. Once you stop smoking, your risk for heart disease can be cut in half in just one year, and the risk continues to decline thereafter. (See Appendix II)

While marriage largely reduces heart disease risk in men, the stress of marriage increases heart disease risk in women.

Stressed – Desserts

These two words are mirror images of each other.

> Stress simply is not taken seriously enough as a
> health threat. No matter what the source of your
> stress, too much of it can increase your risk of
> heart disease.

Chronic stress (stress that you experience over a long time) can result in unhealthy habits which increase your risk of heart disease. Some examples are smoking, lack of regular physical activity, overuse of alcohol, and poor eating habits.

How stress affects your heart

Well, it starts with the unconscious part of the nervous system, called the *autonomic* nervous system. This system has two branches, the sympathetic and parasympathetic. These branches work together to control some of the involuntary activities of the body by producing chemicals that direct those activities. The sympathetic branch normally releases a stress hormone called adrenaline. During stressful moments, a lot of adrenaline is produced in excess which causes your heart rate and blood pressure to soar and stimulates your blood clotting cells called platelets. Most people have felt palpitations at times (a strong heartbeat, racing, or like butterflies on your chest). These indicate an increase in blood pressure and result from increased adrenaline.

When stress continues without letting up over a long period of time, your blood pressure stays higher than normal, and you may develop high blood pressure (hypertension). Stress hormones like adrenaline can damage blood vessels by reducing their flexibility and making them more vulnerable to plaque rupture.

Emotional and mental stress has also been linked with a reduced blood flow to the heart muscle. These appear to be related to tightening of the coronary arteries, especially the smaller ones. This can lead to Coronary microvascular dysfunction (CMD) which is more common in women. This reduced blood flow triggered by stress has been associated with a doubling of risk for future heart attack and death in people with heart disease.

How do you know if you have too much stress?

If you are experiencing too much:

- anger
- back pain
- chest tightness
- headaches
- heart palpitations
- inability to relax at night
- inability to concentrate
- increase in blood pressure
- diagnosed with irritable bowel syndrome
- diagnosed with anxiety or depression

then you probably have an unhealthy amount of stress in your life right now.

Stress from inadequate social and economic resources, being a caregiver, your marriage, and adversities early in life are very common in women. They have also been linked to adverse heart conditions.

Research shows that these factors affect women differently than men. For example, while marriage largely reduces heart disease risk in men, the stress of marriage increases heart disease risk in women.

Studies are needed to better understand the roles these lifestyle risk factors play in women, how to manage them, and how they impact the onset and outcome of heart disease.

Be social

Loneliness appears to be a risk factor for heart disease based on a recent review of studies lead by Dr. N. Valtorta and published in the medical journal *Heart*. This review of multiple studies linked poor social relationships with a 29 percent increase in risk of heart disease. Having a stronger social network appears to benefit your heart.

Further research is needed to assess how these risk factors impact women with heart disease versus men.

I believe that all women would benefit from a better understanding of the associations between reproductive hormones, cardiovascular health, and hormone therapy risk, and get guidance regarding appropriate actions to take to protect their heart health. Together we can advocate for more research to understand this important aspect of our health.

What tests do I need to find out if I have heart disease?

Whether you go to your doctor because you recognize that you have been experiencing symptoms that suggest heart disease, or because you realize that you are at risk, once your doctor completes a history and physical exam she or he might want to do some tests. This all will depend on your symptoms.

Both women and men have heart attacks, but the standard methods for assessing risk for heart disease have not been as effective in women as in men. Approximately 64 percent of women who die suddenly of heart disease had no previous symptoms. This means that traditional risk factors and scores underestimate heart disease risk in women. Therefore, finding more efficient and accurate ways to identify heart disease risk in women is essential.

Tests to diagnose heart disease are less accurate in women than they are in men. Although the American College of Cardiology (ACC) and the American Heart Association (AHA) recommend a stress test as the initial diagnostic test for heart disease, it is less accurate for women.

The current test to detect heart disease focuses on detecting plaque buildup in the coronary arteries that supply the heart with oxygen and nutrients. But women are less likely to have obstructions in the blood flow for the heart muscle. Therefore, the best diagnostic test is one that can identify a lack of blood flow to the heart and its cause. CMD (coronary microvascular dysfunction) is difficult to diagnose as there is no direct test for it.

The great news is that a new study showed that the Cardiac MRI stress T1 test may be an effective way of diagnosing heart disease in women and we hope it will be available to the community in the near future. More research is needed to determine the most efficient and accurate ways of detecting heart disease in women.

Stress test

There are different types of stress tests. The one that the majority of people know is the Exercise Treadmill Test (ETT). During an ETT you walk or run on a treadmill or pedal on a stationary bike while your doctor monitors blood pressure, heart rate, and your heart electrical activity for changes that suggests a blockage of blood flow to the heart.

In some cases, the ETT may be combined with tests (e.g., echocardiogram, single-photon emission computed tomography (SPECT), myocardial perfusion imaging, and cardiac positron emission tomography (PET)) that provide images of your heart showing how the blood is flowing, and how the heart is pumping at rest and stress.

If you cannot walk, then your doctor might suggest a stress test using medications instead. In this type of test, you will not walk on a treadmill, but they will inject a medication into your vein that mimics the effects of exercise.

When your doctor orders this type of test she or he is interested in looking at whether your symptoms may be caused by a blocked artery.

If you have an abnormal stress test your doctor might suggest further testing this time to take a look at your heart arteries and assess the degree of blockage. Among these studies are a computed tomography angiography (CTA) and coronary angiography also known as heart catheterization.

CT scanning of the coronary arteries

A CT scan (computed tomography) uses a number of x-rays to take pictures inside the body. This can also be used to see whether the coronary arteries that supply blood to the heart tissue are blocked.

Results from CT scans appear to have a 26 percent false positive results, indicating that there is a significant blockage or obstruction when in reality there is not. It appears that an explanation to that issue is the amount of calcified plaque as a possible artifact. The presence of severe calcification in the coronary arteries, may tend to appear larger than they really are. In those cases, the blockage appears worse than in reality. The older you are, the higher the chances of having a false positive result with a CT scan (where the scan sees you have a blockage when one doesn't actually exist). Talk to your doctor about whether a CT scan would be helpful or accurate to help determine your heart disease risk.

Heart (or Coronary) Catheterization

This procedure also uses x-rays to see your heart's blood vessels and look for any restrictions in blood flow going to the heart. A coronary angiogram is the most common type of cardiac catheterization used to diagnose and treat heart and blood vessel conditions.

During a coronary angiogram, a type of dye that's visible by an x-ray machine is injected into the blood vessels of your heart. The x-ray machine rapidly takes a series of images to look at the flow in your blood vessels. If necessary, your doctor can open clogged heart arteries performing an angioplasty during that procedure.

Test results

Once your tests are completed you will have your diagnosis and a treatment plan, but unfortunately for many of you, the investigation will end here and you will continue without an explanation for your symptoms.

Angioplasty: A procedure to open blocked arteries on your heart. A thin tube is threaded into your arteries with a small balloon and a stent. Once in the area that is clogged or narrowed, the balloon is inflated opening the obstruction and a stent can be inserted.

Stent: A small metal cylinder that is inserted inside an artery to release a blockage due to plaque.

Approximately 64 percent of women who die suddenly of heart disease had no previous symptoms.

Symptoms of Heart Disease

How many times have you heard this from people: "They did the tests and everything came back normal, but I don't feel good and continue to experience the same symptoms."

My results are normal compared to what?

"We must come to grips with the fact that a 'clean' angiogram in a woman with symptoms does not mean she has a healthy heart."

--Dr. Nitza Alvarez

There are fundamental differences in the blood vessels of women and men that contribute to differences in how heart disease develops, progresses, and responds to treatment. Up to half of people who undergo non-urgent coronary angiograms because of chest pain are found to have no evidence of blocked arteries, however these women had disabling signs and symptoms and long-term adverse events.

Chest pain

The mechanism for chest pain is different for women than for men. In order to understand the different mechanisms, I want you to visualize your coronary circulation like a tree. Your major coronary arteries will be the trunk and there will be multiple branches that get smaller. The smallest branches of all are along the outside of the tree. These branches represent the microvasculature ("micro" for small).

Your chest pain can come from a condition that affects either the main branches of the coronary arteries or the microvasculature. If your chest pain comes from the main branches, this is known as *Vasospastic disease*, a fancy word to describe spasm of your arteries. If the spasm happens once in a while, this will cause a condition known as *Prinzmetal angina*. However, if the spasms are persistent, this can cause a heart attack.

In the last 30 years there have been a number of studies showing that chest pain can be caused by lack of blood flow to the heart from dysfunction of the microvasculature. This condition is known as coronary microvascular dysfunction (CMD). We think that this is the result of both:

1.   Impaired microvascular dilatation, when those small vessels can't relax properly.

2.   Increased microvascular constriction, which involves spasms of these very small arteries. Microvascular constriction can reduce blood flow to the heart muscle enough to cause broken heart syndrome (also known as *Takotsubo syndrome*).

People with microvascular disease are typically female, younger than the usual age for heart disease, and postmenopausal. Chest pain may occur during physical activity or at rest. Symptoms of chest pain may last for hours and there may be flares over a short time period. Because there are a few different causes, not all people find relief from common medications. More than half of people are not helped with the usual medications prescribed to treat chest pain, for example such as nitroglycerin.

A sign that may indicate microvascular disease is chest pain that develops during:

- chemical stress test
- emotional stress
- smoking
- exposure to extreme cold weather.

MINOCA and INOCA

These are terms used to describe when a person, usually a woman, has a heart attack or symptoms of lack of blood flow (also referred to as ischemia), but has no evidence of blocked arteries on an angiogram.

MINOCA is the acronym for: myocardial infarction with no obstructive coronary artery disease. MINOCA represents up to 14 percent of all heart attacks, and it is present more frequently in younger patients.

INOCA is the acronym for: ischemia with non-obstructive coronary artery disease. If you have this condition you will be prescribed medications as well as changes to your lifestyle. The recommended medications include the use of beta-blockers (e.g., atenolol, carvelidol, metoprolol), calcium channel blockers (e.g., amlodipine, Cardiazem®), nitrates (e.g., isosorbide), statins and ACE inhibitors (e.g., benazepril, captopril, lisinopril). Supplements such as L-arginine and pain modulator agents may also be recommended if needed.

> You are not at lower risk of having a heart attack or dying just because your arteries are "normal"

Do not remain silent

Silence about your symptoms might cost you your life, and nobody wants the eternal silence. So please, speak up! If you are describing your symptoms and concerns and you are not heard, speak louder and insist. However, if you continue to be ignored, then it is time to seek medical attention from a different doctor, somebody that is sensitive to your needs, understands that women's symptoms are different, and is capable of recognizing this.

Yes, what you read is what I said: Change your doctor if that is what it takes for you to receive the care that you deserve.

This book is intended to promote awareness of the increased risk that we as women have of dying from a medical condition that is preventable.

What if I exercise?

To my active crew out there: Just because you are active, you are not exempt from heart disease.

Remember from the quiz that sedentary life is only one risk factor. Even when you think that everything is good, it might not be. In my practice, I see a lot of very active patients of all ages. For the most part, when you encounter somebody that exercises routinely, they feel that the words *heart disease* doesn't apply to them. Although exercise will take away one of the risk factors and it will help to control others such as high blood pressure, diabetes, and high blood lipids, it will be important to be examined for subtle symptoms that you might be ignoring, such as mild shortness of breath or fatigue.

Let me share with you the story of one of my beloved patients that came to me because her husband thought that she should see me at least once for a checkup. He said: "She is healthy but, of course, we are getting old." His wife was a very active woman. Her exercise routine consisted of daily running, yoga three times per week, and Pilates 2-3 times per week. She had a healthy diet, mostly consisting of plant-based foods.

On our first visit we started talking about her life. As I inquired about her ability to complete her daily tasks like fixing her bed, gardening, and cleaning, she mentioned that she has been noticing mild shortness of breath while running; but other than that, nothing else. On further questioning she revealed that this shortness of breath is new and has been bothering her, but she thought that it might be her age. I recommended that she do an exercise treadmill test (stress test).

To make a long story short, she had a very abnormal stress test, requiring further testing that revealed severe heart disease requiring intervention as she showed signs of injury to her heart.

Nobody is exempt!

Now, two months later when she goes for her morning run, she is no longer short of breath.

Imagine what would happen if she continued to run and ignore those symptoms?

"We must come to grips with the fact that a 'clean' angiogram in a woman with symptoms does not mean she has a healthy heart."

--Dr. Nitza Alvarez

How can I tell if it's a heart attack?

How can you tell if you or a woman that you love might be experiencing a heart attack or symptoms that suggest CAD (coronary artery disease), such as angina? Even though heart attacks are usually the result of years or decades of heart disease, it may have gone unnoticed until now. It is possible that a heart attack is the first sign that something is wrong with your heart. Recognizing these symptoms might make a difference for your survival.

A heart attack happens when your heart does not receive

> The word "angina" comes from the Greek word ankhone, meaning "strangling." It's a type of chest pain or discomfort caused by reduced blood flow to the heart.

appropriate blood flow through the coronary arteries and it gets injured. This injury results in an inefficient heart; a weak pump. But it can also become a life-threatening condition and even cause death when the injury is large enough to affect the normal function of your heart, like its beat.

What are women's symptoms of a heart attack?
In general, many symptoms of heart attacks in women are referred to as *atypical* symptoms. There is nothing atypical about women's heart attack symptoms other than they are

not the symptoms that are typically experienced by men. It's time that we recognize the differences between women's and men's heart health. Women and men with CAD experience different symptoms and are often treated differently and have different outcomes.

Women should look for symptoms of:

- shortness of breath at rest or during your everyday activities
- abdominal (belly) pressure or discomfort
- lower chest discomfort
- fatigue
- back pain (e.g., pain between your shoulder blades--remember Mrs. N.?)
- nausea

Other classic or *typical* warning signs of heart attack that are more often seen in men but can appear in women include a squeezing feeling in the center of the chest that spreads towards the neck, jaw and shoulder, and chest discomfort associated with nausea, fainting, sweating, and shortness of breath.

As you can see, the most common symptoms of CAD in women can be very subtle and can create a confusing picture which may delay an accurate diagnosis. For many women, this results in many and repeated non-heart-related tests before getting to a definitive diagnosis. This can bring along with it increased worry, sadness, and frustration.

You have to be your own advocate! Unless you are paying attention to your symptoms and insist on getting a medical examination, your heart condition can go undiagnosed and, in the worst-case scenario, result in a heart attack.

If you are experiencing any of the symptoms mentioned above don't hesitate to seek medical attention. If you feel you are not being taken seriously, find another doctor.

Women's poorer health outcomes

Women develop symptoms related to CAD later in life compared to men. About 10 years later. At all ages the presence of CAD is lower among women than men and, despite less plaque buildup in their coronary arteries, women have a higher chance of developing complications and dying from CAD than men. Although knowledge of sex-specific differences has improved, women under the age of fifty are still three times more likely than men to die after a heart attack. Women are significantly less likely to received pharmaceutical and other therapies, such as clot-busting medications or stents, compared to men when they show symptoms of a heart attack.

Research suggests that poorer outcomes may be due to women's hesitancy to seek medical care for their symptoms or not recognizing *atypical* symptoms. When women do seek care, they are also more likely than men to have substantial heart health risks, such as high blood pressure, high bad cholesterol levels, high blood sugar, and depression (yes, depression is a risk factor for heart attacks!).

Another potential explanation for women's poorer outcomes is the differences in the structure and function of some of the blood vessels. The very tiny blood vessels–the *micro*vasculature--may play a greater role in supplying blood to the heart and are more likely to be dysfunctional in women than men.

The experience many women have after seeking care for signs and symptoms of heart disease is that they feel that their doctors dismissed or trivialized their symptoms. These experiences lead to delay in getting an accurate diagnosis. They also lead women to be more hesitant to continue repeating their symptoms to their doctors.

> Please *never* forget that even subtle symptoms count!

If you don't want to be another statistic don't let this behavior stop you. Be your own advocate and don't stop until you get an answer. Even if this requires finding another doctor. If you are not experiencing any symptoms but you know that you are at risk for heart disease, you should also be examined. Prevention is the most important intervention.

PreventTheStent

What are women's risk factors for a heart attack?

Some women don't have any of the traditional risk factors mentioned above and yet still have a heart attack. How do we explain this and what are other risk factors that might contribute to this increased risk?

Numerous research studies have shown that the original traditional risk score, also known as Framingham Risk Score, failed to identify risk in a large number of women. Even up to age eight, more than three out of every four women are considered low risk by this traditional risk score. Today, we understand that CAD goes beyond cholesterol levels and there are some other risk factors that are thought to be associated with an increased risk of heart attack. The reason for this book is to learn about all of the heart disease risk factors that might affect you as a woman.

Women under the age of fifty are still three times more likely than men to die after a heart attack.

What can I do to prevent a heart attack?

To prevent a heart attack, know your risk factors and make sure that you take care of those conditions that require treatment.

- Listen to your doctor's recommendations.
- Be physically active.
- Follow a heart healthy diet.

Physical activity

The American Heart Association (AHA) recommends exercising at least 150 minutes per week of moderate-intensity aerobic activity--that's 30 minutes per day, five days per week. Physical activity is any activity where you move your body and burn calories. The alternative to this is to exercise at least 25 minutes of vigorous aerobic activity 3 days per week for a total of 75 minutes.

Aerobic exercise benefits your heart and includes walking, jogging, swimming, or biking, among others. Strength and stretching exercises are best for overall stamina and flexibility.

Eating habits

Diet plays a crucial part in prevention and treatment of heart disease. However, even among the experts, there is no clear consensus on what is the most appropriate diet to follow to prevent heart disease.

A great example and a good guide is a recent article from 2017: Trending Cardiovascular Nutrition Controversies, published in the *Journal of the American College of Cardiology*. This article focuses on heart health promotion. The consensus is that the future health of the global population largely depends on a shift to eating healthier food. It can be very complicated to develop a dietary plan with all the conflicting information and food available at the stores, many of which claim miraculous benefits. I would like to share with you a few trends that appear to be good starting points. They are backed up with evidence supporting their heart benefits.

Eat more plants

Recently a large study showed a link between animal versus plant intake and death. The evidence suggests that a diet that is mostly plant-based improves risk factors for heart disease and reduces progression of heart disease. This means that eating mainly plants can not *only* reduce your risk of getting heart disease in the first place, but if you have been diagnosed already, a plant-based diet can prevent it from getting worse!

Some examples of heart-healthy plant-based foods include: nuts, olive oil, green leafy vegetables, legumes, and antioxidant-rich foods like colorful vegetables.

On the other hand, a high animal protein intake including processed and unprocessed red meat showed an increase in the number of deaths. These foods are known for being rich in saturated fat. Some examples of products that are high in saturated fats (i.e., are *not* so heart-healthy) are: red meat, chicken skin, ham, mayonnaise, cheese, and dairy products.

To improve your heart-healthy diet eat more protein-rich plants like nuts and legumes and reduce your intake of meat

Fat Facts

There are many different kinds of fats that we eat in our diet. They include saturated fats, trans fats, and several kinds of unsaturated fats.

Saturated and trans fats (not heart-healthy)
When we talk about fats we cannot get away without understanding something known as saturation. Saturated fats occur naturally in many foods and tend to be solid at

room temperature, like butter or the fat in meat. They come mainly from animal sources, including meat and dairy products.

Trans fats are the unhealthiest of all fats. These are man-made and are formed when food manufacturers modify liquid fats (plant oils) to make them solid fats. The chemical process is called partial hydrogenation and adds hydrogen onto liquid oil molecules to form hard margarine or shortening.

Food such as French fries, doughnuts, cakes, cookies, crackers, and other baked goods that are prepared with shortening are high in trans-fat.

High levels of trans fat in the diet are linked with elevated *bad* cholesterol (LDL) and low levels of *good* cholesterol (HDL).

If you limit the amount of trans fat you eat you will help reduce your chance of clogged arteries. There are no guidelines for daily limits, nor any safe daily level of trans fat intake. This means we should eat as little as possible.

Be careful when reading your food labels. Be wise. If you see shortening or partially hydrogenated oil as one of the first ingredients, that product has a lot of unhealthy trans-fat. (See Appendix II for resources on understanding food nutrition labels.)

Do your calculation from the Nutrition Facts Table: Add polyunsaturated and monounsaturated fats to saturated fats and subtract that number from the *Total fat* listed on the label. The answer is the amount of trans fat in the product.

Animal saturated fats and trans fats are not considered good fats for your heart.

Unsaturated fats (heart-healthy)
Unsaturated fats, like mono- or poly-unsaturated fats, tend to be liquid at room temperature (i.e., plant oils).

Monounsaturated fatty acids (MUFAs) protect against heart disease by reducing your LDL while increasing your HDL. This type of fat is good for you if eaten in moderate amounts and is found in plant foods such as nuts, avocados, and vegetable oils (e.g., olive, peanut, canola, sunflower).

The other type of heart-healthy unsaturated fats are the polyunsaturated fatty acids (PUFAs). These come in two types: omega-3 fatty acids and omega-6 fatty acids. Good sources of omega-3 fatty acids are fatty fish such as salmon, mackerel, tuna, herring, and sardines. Good sources of omega-6 fatty acids are walnuts, chia seeds, flax seeds, and sunflower seeds.

Substituting saturated fats (mostly in meat and dairy) for unsaturated fat (mostly in plants) has been associated with prevention of heart disease. The omega-3 PUFAs have other heart-healthy effects like helping to raise your HDL, lower your triglycerides, and are associated with brain health and reduction of inflammation.

Losing weight goes way beyond trying to be pretty.

Overweight and Obesity

Overweight and obesity have reached epidemic proportions here in the United States. According to the most recent National Health and Nutrition Examination Survey, 41.1 percent of women age twenty years and older have obesity which is when your weight is 20 percent or more above normal. Women with obesity have a higher risk of heart attack, even if they have no other risk factors.

Unfortunately, trying to overcome obesity is seen by many as an esthetic issue and some have adopted the position of "staying overweight and loving yourself the way you are." Accepting yourself the way you are is important as we are unique and special; however, this goes beyond the love handles. It's the belly fat in our deeper layers, the one that covers your abdominal organs, that increases your risk of heart disease. This excess internal fat is linked to:

- Cholesterol imbalance (when your HDL goes down, and your LDL goes up).

- High blood sugar levels.

- Increased risk of diabetes (due to resistance to the hormone insulin that helps to lower your blood sugars).

Imagine how much more your heart has to work as your weight increases? Obesity increases the work that your heart has to do in order to deliver the blood to your entire body. Women who are not physically active tend to have more obesity, and are therefore at higher risk of diabetes. They also have lower HDL levels and their vessels are less flexible making them more prone to plaque formation. Losing weight goes way beyond trying to be pretty.

If you claim to love yourself the way you are, but you are not taking care of your body, watching your eating habits, and exercising, then you are not loving yourself.

Can I prevent heart disease with Aspirin®?

Aspirin® has been a mainstay of the primary prevention of heart disease for men since publication of the Physicians Health Study in 1988. That study was conducted on 22,000 predominately white male physicians. However, the use of Aspirin® as a preventive therapy for women was not studied until the Women's Health Study (WHS), published in 2005. The WHS results showed that Aspirin® had no effect on lowering the risk of a heart attack for women.

> The experience many women have after seeking care for signs and symptoms of heart disease is that they feel that their doctors dismissed or trivialized their symptoms.

Emerging risk factors

In 2019 heart disease is still the leading cause of death in America. This statistic reveals that we still don't have a complete understanding of this complex condition. We have been using the traditional risk factors to identify patients at risk for heart disease and despite them, we continue to bury 420,000 women in America every year due to this condition.

For more than a decade now there has been research on novel risk factors and their potential to diagnose heart disease at an early stage. Studies of these emerging risk factors have helped us to understand the complicated process of atherosclerosis and to identify new targets for therapy to prevent heart disease from starting, or slow its progression if you already have it.

Homocysteine

Homocysteine is made by the body's metabolism of an essential amino acid mostly found in animal protein called methionine.

High levels of homocysteine have been linked with damage of artery walls, which can cause plaque buildup.

Who should be checked?

Any woman who has been diagnosed with heart disease but doesn't have traditional risk factors, and any woman who has a family history of early heart disease.

What causes homocysteine levels to go up?

Some of the things that cause homocysteine levels to rise include:

- vitamin B deficiency (vitamins B6, B12, and folate)
- estrogen deficiency
- kidney problems
- organ transplants
- low thyroid hormone levels
- smoking
- stress.

Lowering homocysteine levels reduces your risk for heart disease.

How to lower your homocysteine levels

You can manage this by increasing your dietary intake of B-vitamins:

- Folate (vitamin B9) with more green leafy vegetables, oranges, and fortified cereals. The cereals have folic acid which is a man-made form of folate (but I would rather have you take it in a natural form and avoid processed food).

- Vitamin B6 with bananas, potatoes, bulgur, winter squash, spinach, tofu, chickpeas, tuna, beef liver, salmon, chicken, and turkey breast.
- Vitamin B12 with clams. Clams are by far the richest source of vitamin B12 and beef liver is a close second. Vitamin B12 is also found in salmon, tuna, eggs, milk, yogurt, and cheese.

If you avoid all animal foods you might find it difficult to get enough vitamin B12, as this vitamin is mainly found in animal products, however, some plant foods rich in vitamin B12 include fortified cereals and fortified plant milk.

In order for the B-vitamins to effectively lower homocysteine levels, you need all three: folate, vitamin B6, and vitamin B12. Unfortunately, only a small percentage of Americans get enough B-vitamins from their diet alone. In some cases, taking supplements may be necessary to lower elevated levels of homocysteine. Ask your doctor if you should take a vitamin B supplement.

Lipoprotein(a)

This is a type of lipoprotein that helps transport the cholesterol in the blood, similar to the ones that carry your cholesterol. What makes this *(a)* one different is that it resembles LDL and other particles that promote clotting. It also promotes inflammation and this is not good to have circulating inside your blood vessels. These are why high Lp(a) in the blood is a risk factor for heart disease, atherosclerosis, and blood clots. There are studies showing that this molecule alone is risk factor for heart disease in women.

You should be tested for Lp(a) levels if you have been diagnosed with heart disease but don't have traditional risk factors or if you have family history of early heart disease.

If your level of Lp(a) is 30 mg per dL or higher, your risk for heart disease is higher.

How to lower your Lp(a) levels

Little is known about how to lower Lp(a) levels. Current recommendations are to start with medications to lower LDL if it is elevated. Statins continue to be the recommended therapy because the treatment with statins appears to reduce overall heart disease risks.

Vitamin B3 (niacin) reduces Lp(a) levels by up to 30-40 percent. The recommended dose is 3 g per day.

We still need more research to know the most effective methods of reducing high Lp(a) levels.

C-reactive protein (CRP)

This is a marker of inflammation. Studies have shown that high levels of CRP in women actually predicted their risk of heart attack even when LDL was within range. Sometimes CRP can be elevated years before the first heart attack and is a strong predictor of future heart problems in apparently healthy people. This is important because one-half of heart attacks occur in people who don't have elevated cholesterol.

Inflammation in your body can come from:

- infections (this is one reason why you have heard that dental disease plays a role on cardiovascular disease)

- high cholesterol

- cigarette smoking

- high blood pressure (hypertension)

- diabetes

- colds or sinusitis

- any other high inflammatory state such as arthritis and fibromyalgia.

How to lower your CRP levels

The most effective treatment has been the use of statins and Aspirin®.

Diets high in fiber are associated with lower levels of inflammatory markers. Try eating more foods high in fiber like flax and chia seeds, beans and legumes, whole grains, and nuts.

Consider increasing your intake of the essential mineral magnesium. Most Americans consume magnesium at levels below the recommended amounts. Current dietary guidelines recommend adequate intake of magnesium (310–420 mg per day) in order to maintain health and lower the risk of heart disease. Individuals with intakes below the recommended dietary allowance (RDA) are more likely to have elevated CRP. Foods high in magnesium include nuts and seeds, beans and legumes, whole grains, shellfish and seafood, and leafy greens.

Work with your doctor or dietitian to identify lifestyle and dietary habits that cause inflammation and address them to help in the healing process by reducing the levels of inflammation in your body.

Insulin Resistance

Insulin is the hormone produced by your pancreas (an organ near your stomach) that is key for managing blood sugar. Insulin helps the sugar you absorb from your food get out of your blood and into the cells where it can be used for energy or stored for future use. Glucose is the type of sugar that's the most important source of energy in all organisms. It's the sugar we refer to when we say *blood sugar*. All sugars are a type of carbohydrate.

In a person who has healthy blood sugar levels, eating a typical meal will cause blood glucose levels to go up. These levels activate the pancreas and tell it to produce insulin. Insulin then travels through the body allowing muscles and fat cells to absorb the glucose in the blood to generate energy. As those cells take the glucose out of the blood, the circulating glucose levels go down back to the normal range.

Sometimes the body isn't able to manage blood sugar levels that well. This can be from diabetes or insulin resistance. Insulin resistance is a condition in which a person's body tissues have a lowered response to insulin. It has built up tolerance, or resistance, to the hormone, making it less effective. When this happens, the pancreas will produce even more insulin to make the muscle and fat cells absorb the glucose that they need to continue functioning. With insulin resistance however, blood sugar levels rise despite high levels of insulin. If this is not corrected, your body will continue to produce more insulin until your pancreas can no longer produce enough to overcome the resistance. At that point your glucose levels will remain elevated (prediabetes) and ultimately you can develop type 2 diabetes.

If you have insulin resistance, high blood sugar, increased abdominal obesity, and abnormal cholesterol you are at higher risk of getting heart disease.

The best ways to manage insulin resistance

Diet and physical activity are the best ways to treat insulin resistance before it's too late.

- Physical activity increases the sensitivity of your body to insulin.

- Avoid refined sugars (e.g., white bread, pasta, candy sweets and sugary beverages), and processed food. They tend to cause a spike in blood sugar.

- Choose your food wisely. The amount of carbohydrates in your diet is not as important as the type of carbohydrate. Healthy carbohydrates are those that come from vegetables (caution with potatoes--they are very high in carbohydrates), fruits, beans and whole grain. They are richer in fiber and your body digests fiber slowly, therefore the rise in blood sugar is only moderate avoiding the spikes.

Women under the age of fifty are still three times more likely than men to die after a heart attack.

I Survived!

It is not uncommon to feel frustrated or vulnerable once you find out that you have heart disease. I want you to know that you are not alone. As a specialist in heart diseases in women I see, almost on a daily basis, how my patients seem so vulnerable and sometimes even feel powerless.

If you had a heart attack, allow yourself time to heal. Part of your heart has been injured and needs healing. The post heart attack period is a critical one in which you should be prudent with your physical activity. For the first 6-12 weeks your heart will be going through a lot of changes. You are encouraged to engage in physical activity but this is not the time to try to show off or push yourself to the limit. There is nothing to prove to anybody, nor to yourself.

You will probably need to rest more. Keep in mind that getting enough rest is just as important as taking your medications. Talk to your doctor about a cardiac rehabilitation program. It has been proven to be very effective in the recovery post heart attack.

Talk to your doctor about your feelings. It's common to have a greater awareness of your body at this time. You might even feel like you are too worried about your health, but the best way to get back to your regular routine is communicating all these feelings to your doctor, even if she or he doesn't ask. Your doctor may recommend antidepressants or antianxiety medications to help temporarily.

There are also support groups where you can meet other women with similar medical conditions: Women Heart, the National Coalition for Women with Heart Disease, and Mended Hearts are some examples. These groups do a great job of education, plus you can get tips from other people in the process of recovering from their heart disease.

Returning to work

With the amazing technological improvements in how we can open a blocked artery, and with the medical therapy that we have available to help the heart through the healing process, it will not be necessary for you to stay off work for months like it used to be in the past.

Of course, every case is different depending on the size of the heart attack, the damage to your heart, and complications. Therefore, it will be important to discuss with your doctor and be honest about the type of work that you do so she or he can make an accurate assessment on when it will be appropriate for you to return to work.

The sexy lover

Although some people might require some time before they feel physically or emotionally ready, I can guarantee you that you will not have to restrict yourself from sexual activity for the rest of your life. I know that a heart attack can make you feel very vulnerable, it can make the strongest person feel helpless and frightened.

I once read this quote that summarized it all, "A heart attack acts as reminder of our fragile human nature." Give yourself time. As a rule of thumb if you're able to do moderate exercise (see Appendix III), you are ready to start enjoying your sexual life.

Can I enjoy a drink after a heart attack?

Unfortunately, as far as my investigation went before I wrote this book, there have been no studies that look at this issue in women. However, in France a group of scientists evaluated 353 men who survived and recovered from their first heart attack. They averaged two drinks per day and, apparently, 59 percent were less likely to have additional heart conditions compared to those who abstained from alcohol.

Alcohol has proven to reduce your risk for heart attacks, however in moderation. For women the recommended amount is one drink per day (one drink is one 12 oz. beer, 1 ½ oz. of liquor, or 5 oz. of wine). This is *not* cumulative therefore don't even think about having six or seven drinks at the end of the week for the days that you did not drink during the week.

What about medications?

Heart attacks vary, even among women. Some will have blockage of the certain arteries, while others might have spasms or microvascular disease.

Part of the treatment that your doctor may recommend includes:

- antiplatelet medications
- beta-blockers
- statins
- ACE Inhibitors.

Antiplatelet medications

These medications will help keep the blood flowing and prevent clot formation inside the arteries. A very common one is Aspirin® and, for a certain period of time, you might be given two antiplatelet therapies. The most common side effect of taking these medications is bleeding

Beta-blockers

These medications (e.g., atenolol, carvelidol, metoprolol) are prescribed after a heart attack primarily to block adrenaline receptors that will otherwise accelerate your heart and increase the demand on it.

The sudden injury to the heart reduces its ability to pump blood properly. Therefore, the body releases substances that make the heart beat faster and will injure the heart further This medication will also control your blood pressure, prevent abnormal heart beats, worsening of the heart attack and prevent adverse remodeling of your heart.

The most common side effects of beta-blockers are fatigue, low heart rate, and lightheadedness which happen if your blood pressure is too low.

Statins

These cholesterol medications are part of a big group used for management of high LDL (*bad* cholesterol). They have been around for more than a few decades with a lot of research on how they reduce the number of heart attacks in people with history of heart disease or are at high risk for heart disease. Even when your cholesterol numbers are normal, your doctor might suggest statins after a recent heart attack or stent.

Statins lower the amount of LDL in the blood by reducing the production of cholesterol in the liver. Some of the statins include atorvastatin (Lipitor®), fluvastatin (LEscol®), lovastatin (Mevacor®), pitavastatin (Livalo®), pravastatin (Pravachol®) rosuvastatin (Crestor®), and simvastatin (Zocor®).

The new cholesterol guidelines recommend that statins be prescribed to individuals with:

- a history of prior heart attack, stroke, or angina
- high LDL >190 mg per dL, despite risk
- a high risk of having a heart attack in the next 10 years
- diabetes between the ages of forty and seventy-five.

Atherosclerosis goes beyond your cholesterol numbers and is much more complex. In addition to lowering your cholesterol, statins help to reduce inflammation and stabilize and reduce the plaque that is already inside your vessels. The less stable the plaque, the more likely it is to break apart or rupture and cause a heart attack.

Even if your heart attack was caused by microvascular disease (which is the main difference between women and men with CAD), there are studies to suggest that patients with microvascular disease benefit from the use of statins. In studies of these patients, statin therapy improved function of the lining of the blood vessels and reduced or eliminated limited blood flow to the heart. Therefore, statin therapy might play a role in the treatment of microvascular angina.

The most common side effects of statins are muscle pain and it may affect the liver

ACE inhibitors

A heart attack results from reduced oxygen supply (ischemia) to a small section of the heart and heart damage. When this happens, the body wants to remodel, but what we want is for the heart muscle to heal. ACE inhibitors are proven to reduce the chances of remodeling and help the heart to heal. These medications have been shown to improve long-term survival after a heart attack and reduce the risk for another heart attack and sudden death.

ACE inhibitors, like beta-blockers, are considered a must after a heart attack.

The most common side effect of ACE inhibitors is cough.

The most common symptoms of CAD in women can be very subtle and can create a confusing picture which may delay an accurate diagnosis.

Heart Failure in Women

When we think about heart disease, heart attack normally comes to mind. We are less likely to think of heart failure as a cardiovascular catastrophe even though it affects more than three million women, is the leading reason for hospitalization, and a major cause of death in women over sixty-five years old.

Heart failure, like coronary artery disease, may be different in women as we tend to suffer more from diastolic heart failure rather than systolic heart failure. (weakening of the heart).

I cannot breathe, what can that be?

Many women experience shortness of breath as they age. Are you having hard time completing your daily tasks? Do you keep running out of breath despite "normal" results? These symptoms might have been attributed to many things, but not your heart.

Diastolic dysfunction (stiff heart)

As you get older, especially after menopause, there is a common condition seen in women called *diastolic dysfunction* which is a medical term to explain a stiff heart. Stiffness of the heart can be the explanation for your difficulty breathing as you are completing chores in the house, walking through the grocery store, making your bed, or practicing your favorite sport with your friends. If you notice that you get winded easily with your activities and this is something new to you, this condition might be the reason for your symptoms.

Diastolic dysfunction happens as a consequence of your heart not relaxing well. When your heart does not relax well it gets stiff. Less blood can enter a stiff chamber, so some of it flows backwards to your lungs.

When this happens, some blood accumulates in your lungs where there is supposed to be air. This is called *pulmonary congestion*, often referred to as fluid or water in the lungs. When there is water in your lungs you cannot breathe normally and it may feel a bit like drowning. This is what makes you feel short of breath.

When you are resting and your body is not demanding too much oxygen you might not feel short of breath. However, as soon as you start moving and the demand increases you will have difficulty breathing. As you move around, your heart beats faster and this is why you feel short of breath when you move. If your heart is stiff, it will be even harder to do its job pumping blood when it needs to beat faster. The faster the heartbeat, the less time it has to relax between beats.

Causes of a stiff heart

One of the most common causes for this condition is high blood pressure. Other causes include:

- obesity
- diabetes
- lung conditions such as chronic obstructive pulmonary disease (COPD)
- anemia
- kidney conditions, like chronic renal insufficiency (CRI) (where there is gradual loss of kidney function).

All these conditions cause inflammation in the body and, as a consequence, promotes the production of substances in your system that promote stiffening of your heart and arteries.

Limitations in the production of nitric oxide (NO) is commonly seen in post-menopausal women and it is another common cause of this condition. Nitric oxide is a compound produced by the lining of the interior wall of the arteries. It helps widen the blood vessels.

New studies suggest that diastolic dysfunction might be directly related to coronary microvascular dysfunction (CMD). The injury that this condition causes to your heart will contribute to remodeling of the chambers of the heart that serve as the pump, making it difficult for them to relax. The formation of remodeling tissue and stiffness of the arteries also contributes to the stiffness of the heart.

How is a stiff heart diagnosed?

The most common way to diagnose a stiff heart is to do an ultrasound of your heart, called an echocardiogram. This is similar to the ultrasounds that they do on expectant mothers to see the baby, but instead of a baby we look at your heart. This test is very safe because it is non-invasive, free of radiation, and uses high frequency sound waves instead.

Through the echocardiogram we can evaluate the different phases of heart function including its ability to relax and the severity of the stiffness, among other things. Without an echocardiogram it is difficult to know if diastolic dysfunction is present and it might go undiagnosed for a long time while you continue feeling short of breath.

Sometimes your doctors will not even think about diastolic function as a possible cause for your shortness of breath. Thus, if you have been experiencing difficulty breathing and they have still not found the reason, or if they perhaps found a possible cause but despite treatment you are still short of breath, discuss with your doctor your concerns about stiff heart.

Is there any treatment for stiff heart?

Once you develop a stiff heart, the most important steps to follow are to treat your high blood pressure, reduce your inflammation, and use medication to get rid of the excess of water if you are experiencing symptoms of shortness of breath.

I suggest the use of the supplement L-arginine to promote nitric oxide production because it has shown to improve relaxation of your heart muscle. If you have a stiff heart but you have no symptoms, perhaps supplementing your body to naturally increase the production of relaxers is not a bad idea.

Does everybody with a stiff heart have shortness of breath?

No. You can have a stiff heart and be absolutely symptom free.

Heart failure

When you experience difficulty breathing and your doctor finds that you have a stiff heart with signs of water retention, this is called heart failure. This statement means that your heart *is failing.* It is failing to complete its task: to pump blood. It is pumping inefficiently because it can't fill properly. The blood backs up into the circulation of the lungs and causes congestion. This type of heart failure affects about 3.6 million women in the United States.

Treatment for heart failure

If you have been diagnosed with heart failure your doctor will recommend a medication to alleviate your symptoms by reducing water retention in your lungs. These medications are call diuretics.

Other medications may include one to lower your heart rate (if you have a fast one), and another if you have a thick heart.

You may be wondering if, with excess water in your lungs, you should drink less fluids. There is a very fine line between water retention and dehydration with this condition, therefore make sure that you keep yourself hydrated. Remember that fluid restriction is not going to make your heart relax any better but it will prevent excess fluid on it. In fact, it is more important to limit your salt intake.

Despite the fact that women account for nearly 50 percent of all hospital admission for heart failure, only 25 percent of people who participate in heart failure studies are women.

Palpitations? Fluttering?

The electrical system of your heart

Your heart is a pump that needs electricity! There is an electrical pulse that makes the heart muscle contract and pump the blood. Every heart beat starts with an electrical impulse. Whenever the electrical impulses in the heart don't work well, this can cause problems known as arrhythmias. An arrhythmia is a disturbance of a normal heart beat.

Some examples of arrhythmias include:

- Bradycardia (low pulse).
- Conduction disorders (heart block): This happens when the electricity travels through the heart intermittently. For better understanding of this condition I want you to imagine an electrical cord with partial broken wires in which sometimes you have to manipulate the wires to help the electricity travel thru them.
- Tachycardia (rapid pulse).

Tachycardia is a big bucket that includes:

- SVT (supraventricular tachycardia): Rapid pulse coming from the upper chambers of your heart (the atria).

- Premature contractions: A premature beat causes your heart to beat early before the next regular heartbeat. They can go unnoticed but some patients experience palpitations, dizziness, and lightheadedness. Some others experience a strong heartbeat and sometimes the sensation that the heart stop beating momentarily.

- Atrial fibrillation (AF): In this type of arrhythmia the heartbeat that originates in the upper chambers of the heart is irregular, unorganized and rapid. This make the upper chambers of the heart quiver instead of beating effectively.

- Atrial flutter: A more organized arrhythmia that originates in the atrium. Although treated similarly to atrial fibrillation, in this condition the heartbeat appears more organized.

- Ventricular tachycardia: Originates in the ventricle. Mostly seen in women with heart disease. The treatment varies and it depends on symptoms and other medical conditions. This is considered a serious rhythm problem that can become a life-threatening problem. This arrhythmia requires immediate attention.

Chambers of the heart (atria and ventricles): *Within the heart lie four hollow chambers, two atria and two ventricles. The right and left atria serve as volume reservoir for blood that will be send to the ventricles. The ventricles serve as pumping chambers of the heart.*

Is my condition an electrical problem?

If you experience palpitations, dizzy spells, and/or shortness of breath with physical activity, your doctor will recommend these tests:

1. Electrocardiogram (ECG): The 12-lead ECG is a commonly used diagnostic tool. This uses a series of electrodes placed on the person's arms, legs, and chest wall to assess the heart activity from 12 different views.

2. A monitor (if the electrocardiogram does not show any disorder). This monitoring system records the heart's electrical activity as the person follows her normal routine. You will wear a small electronic recorder. This is used to identify intermittent heart rhythm disturbances known as arrhythmias. There are a few different kinds of monitors:

   2.1. Holter monitor: 24-48-hour monitor

   2.2. 30-day monitor: this might be useful if your symptoms don't happen every day.

   2.3. Loop recorders: Implantable monitor. Your doctor will recommend this if the other monitors did not show anything and the rest of the work-up has been negative but you continue to experience your symptoms.

3. Echocardiogram to evaluate the structure of the heart. It shows abnormalities of the heart.
4. A stress test might be recommended to see if your arrhythmia is triggered by exercise.

Once your doctor identifies the type of arrhythmia you have, she or he will recommend a treatment. This might include lifestyle changes such as limiting alcohol, caffeinated beverages, and ensuring proper hydration; taking medications; and sometimes a procedure to treat your rhythm problem.

Of all of these electrical problems of the heart, I want to elaborate on atrial fibrillation, as this is another area where gender differences have been recognized (even though it has received less attention than heart attack).

Atrial fibrillation (AF)
Atrial fibrillation is the most common arrhythmia worldwide. Women with AF have a higher risk of death compared to men with AF. Atrial fibrillation has even been shown to be a risk factor for dementia.

Studies indicate that among people with AF, women are more likely than men to experience symptoms. Moreover, in women AF is associated with worse symptoms and quality of life, and increased risk of complications.

Classical symptoms of AF are heart palpitations, shortness of breath, dizziness, and chest pain. There are some atypical symptoms such as weakness and fatigue.

If your symptoms are not considered typical, then this might contribute to the worse outcomes seen in women. This is because it often provokes a delay in seeking medical attention, and that delay increases the risk.

What's my stroke risk if I have AF?

Even though it is a risk for stroke, little is known of the underlying mechanism. The AHA and The American College of Cardiology (ACC) recommend the use of a score known as CHA_2DS_2-Vasc Score to predict your stroke risk and offer guidance on anticoagulation therapy.

CHA$_2$DS$_2$-Vasc Score

Give yourself one point for each condition that you might have:

- Heart failure _____
- Hypertension _____
- Older than sixty-five years _____
  (two points if older than seventy-five years)
- Diabetes _____
- Vascular disease _____
  (prior heart attack, atherosclerosis, or PVD)
- Female ____
- Stroke ____ (two points)

If you have AF and your CHA$_2$DS$_2$-Vasc Score is two or greater than two, you are at risk for stroke; therefore, a medication that helps prevent blood from clotting is recommended. Aspirin® and other antiplatelet therapies are not the right choice to prevent stroke if you have AF. Talk to your doctor about alternatives of therapy, these medications include: vitamin K antagonists (e.g. Warfarin) and all the new Novel Oral Anticoagulants (NOAC's) such as Apixaban (Eliquis®), dabigatran (Pradaxa®), edoxaban (Savaysa®), rivaroxaban (Xarelto®).

Atrial fibrillation was found to be an independent risk factor for new-onset heart failure with preserved ejection fraction (HfpEf) in women, but not in men. Studies have established the association between AF and risk of a heart attack showing that AF is associated with a two-fold higher risk of heart attack.

Risk factors for AF

Risk factors for atrial fibrillation include: age, and existing heart condition such as valvular disease, heart failure, high blood pressure, coronary artery disease (CAD), diabetes, and obesity.

Although the mechanisms how AF occurs has been studied extensively through the years, our understanding of the differences in heart anatomy in women vs. men, and how the hormones contribute to risk and outcome of AF is insufficient therefore this should be evaluated more. Future research is needed to address the knowledge gaps in sex differences in AF.

Heart valves: The heart contains four valves. The valves allow forward flow of blood through the heart and prevent backward flow.

The most common symptoms of CAD in women can be very subtle and can create a confusing picture which may delay an accurate diagnosis.

GG – Gender Gap

Despite the efforts to improve diagnosis and treatment of heart disease in women, we still encounter significant gaps in understanding how the disease starts and progresses, and how to best treat it. As a specialist in the management of heart disease I believe in working to develop the best tools to be able to identify it before it becomes a life-threatening problem, but more so, *my philosophy is prevention.* Prevention will always be better than treatment.

This book is my initial written effort to spread the word to all women. It is up to us how medical care is going to change in the future. Once you are able to recognize your risk factors and symptoms you can be your own advocate, and that day you are working together with many other women in closing that gap.

Every woman's life matters. Some doctors are not aware of the differences, they are not aware of disparities in the care delivered to women (heels) vs. men (ties); or even of the different signs and symptoms of heart disease in women.

With this book I intend to empower you, your daughters, mother, cousins, aunts, neighbors, and friends to take charge of your health and choose life. A healthy life. And I hope it will help you prevent the stent.

#PreventTheStent

References

Ades, P.A., Waldmann, M.L., Polk, D.M., J.T., & Coflesky, J.T. (1992). Referral Patterns and Exercise Response in the Rehabilitation of Female Coronary Patients Aged Greater Than or Equal to 62 Years. American Journal of Cardiology, 69, 1422-1425.

Alexander, K.P., Shaw, L.J., Delong, E.R., et al. (1998). Value of Exercise Treadmill Testing in Women. Journal of the American College of Cardiology, 32(6), 1657-64.

Arad, Y., Spadaro, L.A., Goodman, K., et al. (2000). Prediction of Coronary Events with Electron Beam Computed Tomography. Journal of the American college of Cardiology, 36(4), 1253-60.

Bairey Merz, C.N., Pepine, C.J., Walsh, M.N., & Fleg, J.L. (2017). Ischemia and no obstructive coronary artery disease (INOCA): developing evidence-based therapies and research agenda for the next decade. Circulation, 135, 1075–1092.

Bless, H., Schwarz, N., Clore, G.L., Golisano, V., et al. (1996). Mood and the Use of Scripts: Does a Happy Mood Really Lead to Mindlessness? Journal of Personality and Social Psychology, 71, 665-69.

Centers for Disease Control and Prevention. Current Cigarette Smoking Among Adults—United States, 2016. Morbidity and Mortality Weekly Report 2018, 67(2), 53-9. Accessed February 22, 2018.

Chen, C., Wei, J., AlBadri, A., Zarrini, P., & Bairey Merz, C.N. (2016). Coronary microvascular dysfunction- epidemiology, pathogenesis, prognosis, diagnosis, risk factors and therapy. Circ J, 81, 3-11.

Chugh, S.S., et al. (2014). Worldwide epidemiology of atrial fibrillation: a Global Burden of Disease 2010 Study. Circulation, 129, 837–47.

Cooper, R., Cutler, J., Nickens, P.D., et al. (2000). Trends and Disparities in Coronary Heart Disease, Stroke and other Cardiovascular Disease in the United States. Circulation, 102, 173-178.

de Lonrgeri, M., Samen, P., Martin, J.L., et al. (1999). Mediterranean Diet, Traditional Risk Factors, and the Rate of Cardiovascular Complications After Myocardial Infarction: First Report of the Lyon diet Heart Study. Circulation, 99, 779-85.

Eikelboom, J.W., Lonn, E., Gensest, J., et al. (1999). Homocysteine and Risk for cardiovascular Disease. Annals of Internal Medicine, 131(5), 363-75.

Farley, T.A., Dalal, M.A., Mostashari, F., & Frieden, T.R. (2010). Deaths preventable in the U.S. by improvements in use of clinical preventive services. Am J Prev Med, 38(6), 600-9.

Freeman, A.M., Morris, P.B. ,Barnard, N., Esselstyn, C.B., Ros, E., Agatston, A., Devries, S., O'Keefe, J., Miller, M., Ornish, D., Williams, K., & Kris-Etherton, P. (2017). Trending Cardiovascular Nutrition Controversies. Journal of the American College of Cardiology, 69(9), 1172-1187. doi: 10.1016/j.jacc.2016.10.086

Goldberg, Nieca. *Women are not small men: Life-Saving Strategies for Preventing and Healing Heart Disease in Women.* Ballantine Books, 2002.

Grodsrein, F., Stampfer, M.J., Manson, J.E., et al. (1996). Postmenopausal Estrogen and Progestin Use and the Risk of Cardiovascular Disease. New England Journal of Medicine, 335(7),453-61.

Hanjai, K.J. (1999). Potential New Cardiovascular Risk Factors: Left Ventricular Hypertrophy, Homocysteine, Lipoprotein(a), Triglycerides, Oxidative Stress, and Fibrinogen. Annals of Internal Medicine, 131(5), 376-86.

Holt-Lunstad, J., & Smith, T.B. (2016). Loneliness and social isolation as risk factors for CVD: implications for evidence-based patient care and scientific inquiry. Heart. doi: 10.1136/heartjnl-2015-309242

Humphries, K.H., et al. (2001). New-onset atrial fibrillation: sex differences in presentation, treatment, and outcome. Circulation, 103, 2365–70.

Lagerqvist, B., Safstrom, K., & Stahle, E. (2001). Is Early Invasive Treatment of Unstable Coronary Artery Disease Equally Effective on Men and Women. Journal of the American College of Cardiology, 38, 41-48.

Ledebogen, F., Gilles, M., Mara, A., et al. (2001). Increased Platelet Aggregability in Major Depression? Psychiatry Research, 102(3), 255-61.

Legato, Marianne J. *The Female Heart: : The Truth about Women and Heart Disease.* William Morrow & Company, 2000.

Levy, S., & Crijns, H.J. (2008). Prognosis, disease progression, and treatment of atrial fibrillation patients during 1 year: follow-up of the Euro Heart Survey on atrial fibrillation. Eur Heart J, 29(9), 1181-9. doi: 10.1093/eurheartj/ehn139.

Lloyd-Jones, D.M., et al. (2004). Lifetime Risk for Development of Atrial Fibrillation: The Framingham Heart Study. Circulation, 110, 1042–1046.

Marcus, B. (1999). The Efficacy of Exercise as an Aid for Smoking Cessation in Women: A Randomized Clinical Trial. Archives of Internal Medicine, 159(11), 1229-34.

Mosca, L., Collins, P., Herrington, D.M., et al. (2001). Hormone Replacement Therapy and Cardiovascular Disease: A Statement for Healthcare Professionals from the American Heart Association. Circulation, 104, 499-503.

Mosca, L., et al. (2011). Sex/Gender Differences in Cardiovascular Disease Prevention. What a Difference a Decade Makes. Circulation, 124(19), 2145-54. doi: 10.1161/CIRCULATIONAHA.110.968792.

Mozzafarian, D., Benjamin, E.J., Go, A.S., et al. (2015). Heart Disease and Stroke Statistics-2015 Update: a report from the American Heart Association. Circulation, e29-322.

National Institutes of Health, Office of Dietary Supplements. Vitamin B12 Fact sheet. Accessed February, 2019.

Nieuwlaat, R., Prins, M.H., Le Heuzey, J.Y., Vardas, P.E., Aliot, E., Santini, M., Cobbe, S.M., Widdershoven, J.W., Baur, L.H.,

Orth-Gomer, K., Mittleman, M.A., Schenck-Gustafsson, K., Wamala, S.P., et al. (1997). Lipoprotein(a) as a Determinant of Coronary Heart Disease in Young Women. Circulation, 95, 329-34.

Pacheco, C., Odayme, Q., Pepine, C.J., & Bairey Merz, C.N. (2018). Why names matter for women: MINOCA/INOCA (myocardial infarction/ischemia and no obstructive coronary artery disease). Clinical Cardiology, 41. 10.1002/clc.22894.

Pepine, C.J. (2004). Ischemic Heart Disease in Women: Facts and Wishful Thinking. J Am Coll Cardiol, 43(10), 1727-30.

Pepine, C.J. et al. (2006). Some Thoughts on the Vasculopathy of Women With Ischemic Heart Disease. J Am Coll Cardiol, 7, 47(3 Suppl), S30-5.

Pepine, C.J., Ferdinand, K.C., Shaw, L.J., Light-McGroary, K.A., Shah, R.U., Gulati, M., Duvernoy, C., Walsh, M.N., & Bairey Merz, C.N. (2015). Emergence of nonobstructive coronary artery disease: a woman's problem and need for change in definition on angiography. J Am Coll Cardiol, 66, 1918–1933.

Ridker, P.M., Hennekens, C.H., Buring, J.E., & Rifai, N. (2000). C-reactive Protein and Other Markers of Inflammation in the Prediction of Cardiovascular Disease in Women. New England Journal of Medicine, 342(12), 836-43.

Rosenfeld, A. (2006). State of the Heart: Building Science to Improve Women's Cardiovascular Health. Am J Crit Care, 15(6), 556-66, quiz 567.

Shaw, L.J., Merz, C.N., Pepine, C.J., Reis, S.E., Bittner, V., Kip, K.E., Kelsey, S.F., Olson, M., Johnson, B.D., Mankad, S., Sharaf, B.L., Rogers, W.J., Pohost, G.M. & Sopko, G. (2006). The economic burden of angina in women with suspected ischemic heart disease: results from the National Institutes of Health—National Heart, Lung, and Blood Institute–Sponsored Women's Ischemia Syndrome Evaluation. Circulation, 114, 894–904.

Shah, A.J., et al. (2014). Sex and Age Differences in the Association of Depression With Obstructive Coronary Artery Disease and Adverse Cardiovascular Events. Journal of the American Heart Association: Cardiovascular and Cerebrovascular Disease, 3.3, e000741.

Svennberg, E., et al. (2015). Mass Screening for Untreated Atrial Fibrillation: The STROKESTOP Study. Circulation, 131, 2176–84.

Taqueti, V.R., et al. (2017). Excess Cardiovascular Risk in Women Relative to Men Referred for Coronary Angiography Is Associated with Severely Impaired Coronary Flow Reserve, Not Obstructive Disease. Circulation, 135.6, 566–577.

Taylor, S.E., Klein, L.C., Lewis, B.P., Gruenewald, T.L., Gurung, R.A., & Updegraff, J.A. (2000). Biobehavioral Responses to Stress in Females: Tend-and-Befriend, not Fight-or-Flight. Psychological Review, 107(3), 411-29.

Vaccarino, V., Parsons, L., Every, N.R., Barron, H., et al. (1999). Sex-Based Differences in Early Mortality After Myocardial Infarction. New England Journal of Medicine 341(4), 217-25.

Valtorta, N.K., Kanaan, M., Gilbody, S., Ronzi, S., & Hanratty, B. (2016). Loneliness and social isolation as risk factors for coronary heart disease and stroke: systematic review and meta-analysis of longitudinal observational studies. Heart, 102(13), 1009-16. doi: 10.1136/heartjnl-2015-308790.

Wei, J., Nelson, M.D., Sharif, B., Shufelt, C., & Bairey Merz, C.N. (2018). Why do we care about coronary microvascular dysfunction and heart failure with preserved ejection fraction: addressing knowledge gaps for evidence-based guidelines. European Heart Journal, 39(37), 3451–3453.

Appendix

Appendix I

Food additive	Where is it found? / How is it use?	Harmful effects
Monosodium Glutamate (MSG)	Common food additive used to intensify and enhance the flavor of savory dishes	Associated with weight gain and metabolic syndrome
High-Fructose Corn Syrup	It is a sweetener made from corn. Found in soda, juices, candy and snack foods	Weight gain and diabetes. Increase inflammation
Artificial flavoring	Design to mimic food flavor	Bone marrow suppression when consume in high amounts.
Artificial sweeteners	Added to many die3t foods and beverages to enhance sweetness	Headache and aspartame have been associated with cancer
Sodium Nitrite	Use as preservative to reduce bacteria growth and add the pink color, salty flavor to the food. Found in process meat.	Stomach, colorectal, bladder and breast cancer. Increase incidence of DM Type I
Artificial food coloring	Us to brighten up and improve the appearance of food.	Increase the risk of thyroid tumor (Red 3). Might promote hyperactivity.
Carrageenan - derive from Seaweed	Used as thickener, emulsifier, and preservative. Mostly found on almond milk, cottage cheese, ice cream coffee creamers, and dairy-free products.	Increase levels of fasting blood sugar and glucose intolerance.
Sodium Benzoate	Preservative often added to carbonated drinks and acidic foods (salad dressings, pickles and condiments)	If combined with Vit C it might form Benzene and increase the risk for cancer.
Trans Fat	Found in processed foods like baked goods, margarine, microwave popcorn. Increase shelf life.	Increase inflammation. Associated with development of cardiovascular disease.

Appendix II

Further resources

"Understanding Food Nutrition Labels." American Heart Association (AHA). Last reviewed March 6, 2018, https://www.heart.org/en/healthy-living/healthy-eating/eat-smart/nutrition-basics/understanding-food-nutrition-labels

"Quit Smoking Resources." Centers for Disease Control and Prevention (CDC). Last reviewed Dec 11, 2017, https://www.cdc.gov/tobacco/quit_smoking/how_to_quit/resources/index.htm

Appendix III

Estimated women caloric needs per day by age and physical activity level

Age	Sedentary	Moderately Active	Active
18	1,800	2,000	2,400
19-25	2,000	2,200	2,400
26-30	1,800	2,000	2,400
31-50	1,800	2,000	2,200
51-60	1,600	1,800	2,200
61 and up	1,600	1,800	2,000

Note that these recommendations are to maintain your weight. If weight loss is intended there will be further caloric restrictions.

Source: Institute of Medicine. Dietary Reference intakes for Energy, Carbohydrate, Fiber, Fat, Fatty Acids, Cholesterol, Protein, and Amino Acids. Washington (DC): The National Academies Press; 2002

Sedentary – means a lifestyle that include the physical activity required for daily living.

Moderately Active - means a lifestyle that includes physical activity equivalent to walking about 1.5 to 3 miles per day at 3 to 4 miles per hour in addition to the activity of daily living.

Active- means a lifestyle that includes physical activity equivalent to walking more than 3 miles per day at 3 to 4 miles per hour, in addition to the activities of daily living.

Glossary

Adipose tissue: Fat in the body. The deeper abdominal adipose tissue, the kind you can't see that is around your internal organs, is known as visceral adipose tissue.

Anemia: Having a lower than normal amount of hemoglobin in the blood. Hemoglobin is part of the oxygen-carrying protein inside red blood cells.

Angina: The word "angina" comes from the Greek word ankhone, meaning "strangling." It's a type of chest pain or discomfort caused by reduced blood flow to the heart.

Angiogram: See *cardiac catheterization.*

Angioplasty: A procedure to open blocked arteries on your heart. A thin tube is threaded into your arteries with a small balloon and a stent. Once in the area that is clogged or narrowed, the balloon is inflated opening the obstruction and a stent can be inserted.

Arrhythmia: Irregular heartbeat; a variation in the normal beat of the heart. Atrial fibrillation is the most common arrhythmia worldwide.

Artery: A vessel in which blood flows from the heart to all parts of the body.

Atherosclerosis: The condition where your arteries get plugged with plaque from cholesterol that builds up on the inside walls causing continuous inflammation. It results in a "stiffening" of the arteries.

Atria: See *chambers of the heart.*

Atrial fibrillation: See *arrhythmia.*

Autonomic nervous system: This system has two branches, the sympathetic and parasympathetic. These branches work together to control some of the involuntary activities of the body by producing chemicals that direct those activities. The sympathetic branch normally releases a stress hormone called adrenaline.

Bile: Bile is made by the liver. It is composed of bilirubin, cholesterol, and bile acids and salts.

Blood pressure: See *high blood pressure.*

Blood vessels: Tubes (arteries and veins) through which blood reaches the tissues and organs. The very tiny blood vessels are called the "microvasculature."

Broken heart syndrome: See *Takotsubo syndrome.*

Cardiac catheterization: A procedure that uses x-rays to see your heart's blood vessels and look for any restrictions in blood flow going to the heart. A coronary angiogram is the most common type of cardiac catheterization procedure used to diagnose and treat heart and blood vessel conditions.

Chambers of the heart: Within the heart lie four hollow chambers, two atria and two ventricles. The right and left atria serve as volume reservoir for blood that will be sent to the ventricles. The ventricles serve as pumping chambers of the heart.

Cholesterol: See *lipoprotein.*

Chronic obstructive pulmonary disease (COPD): Long standing inflammatory condition that interferes with normal breathing.

Clot: When some of the blood component clump together, as in a scab that forms when you cut your skin. This is caused by your blood-clotting cells called platelets.

Conduction disorders (heart block): This happens when the electricity travels through the heart intermittently. For better understanding of this condition I want you to imagine an electrical cord with partial broken wires in which sometimes you have to manipulate the wires to help the electricity travel through them.

Coronary angiogram: See *cardiac catheterization*.

Coronary arteries: The arteries located on the heart that supply blood to the heart tissue. They have multiple branches like a tree. The smallest branches of all (along the outside) are called the microvasculature ("micro" for small).

Coronary artery disease (CAD): A disease of the vessels that supply blood to your heart. This is a long-term condition that increases your risk for, and can eventually lead to a heart attack.

Coronary artery dissection: A break in the internal lining of the wall of the arteries causing a quick stop of blood flow to the heart muscle.

Coronary calcium score: Coronary artery calcium scan measures the calcification of your heart arteries helping us to predict a person's risk of heart disease.

Coronary microvascular dysfunction (CMD): Tightening of the small coronary arteries affecting their walls and inner lining. This reduces blood flow to the heart and is triggered by emotional and mental stress. CMD is associated with a doubling of risk for future heart attack and is more common in women. We think that this is the result of both impaired microvascular dilatation (when those small vessels can't relax properly) and increased microvascular constriction (which involves spasms of these very small arteries). New studies suggest that CMD might be directly related to diastolic dysfunction.

C-reactive protein (CRP): A marker of inflammation. Studies have shown that high levels of CRP in women actually predicted their risk of heart attack even when LDL was within range.

CT scan (computed tomography): An imaging test that uses a number of x-rays to take pictures inside the body. This can be used to see whether the coronary arteries that supply blood to the heart tissue are blocked.

Diabetes: A condition where there are high sugar (glucose) levels in your blood. This results from the body's inability to use blood sugar for energy. In Type 1 diabetes, the body no longer makes insulin and therefore blood sugar cannot leave the blood and enter the cells to be used for energy. In Type 2 diabetes, either the body can no longer make enough insulin or the body is unable to use insulin correctly. One of the most severe complications of diabetes is the early onset of plaque and atherosclerosis. When diabetes develops during pregnancy, it's called gestational diabetes.

Diastolic dysfunction: A medical term to explain a stiff heart. Diastolic dysfunction happens as a consequence of your heart not relaxing well. When your heart does not relax well, it gets stiff. New studies suggest that diastolic dysfunction might be directly related to coronary microvascular dysfunction (CMD).

Echocardiogram: A very safe, non-invasive, radiation-free test that uses high-frequency sound waves to do an ultrasound of the heart. Echocardiograms evaluate the structure of the heart, showing abnormalities. It is used to check for arrhythmias and is the most common way to diagnose diastolic dysfunction.

Endothelium: The tissue that forms a single layer of cells lining the blood vessels.

Exercise treadmill test (ETT): See *stress test*.

Gestational diabetes: See *diabetes*.

Glucose: The type of sugar that's the most important source of energy in all organisms. It's the sugar we refer to when we say blood sugar. All sugars are a type of carbohydrate.

Heart attack: When your heart gets injured because it did not receive appropriate blood flow through the coronary arteries. This is also known as "myocardial infarction," or MI, and is often the result of many years living with improperly managed heart disease.

Heart failure (HF): A condition in which the heart doesn't pump blood effectively. Either because it is weak or it cannot fill properly.

Heart rate: Also known as your pulse.

High blood pressure: Also known as hypertension (HTN) or the "silent killer." Blood pressure is the force of the blood pushing against the wall of the blood vessels. When the heart beats the flow of the blood through the arteries pushes with high force over a sustained period of time. Blood pressure has two components: Systolic blood pressure and diastolic blood pressure. The systolic blood pressure is the top number that represents the pressure generated by the heart when it beats to pump blood. Diastolic blood pressure is the bottom blood pressure that represent the pressure in the blood vessels between heart beats. If you have a blood pressure monitor, your blood pressure is elevated if it's higher than 140/90 mmHg. Hypertension is a diagnosis made after consecutive readings with elevated blood pressure.

Homocysteine: Homocysteine is made by the metabolism of an essential amino acid mostly found in animal protein called methionine. High levels of homocysteine have been linked with damage of artery walls, which can cause plaque buildup.

Inflammation: When the body's immune system reacts to infections, wounds or tissue damage. When it occurs for a long time it can eventually lead to several diseases or conditions including plaque formation and stiffening of your heart and arteries.

INOCA: The acronym for: *ischemia with non-obstructive coronary artery disease.*

Insulin: The hormone produced by your pancreas (an organ near your stomach) that is key for managing blood sugar. Insulin helps the sugar you absorb from your food get out of your blood and into the cells where it can be used for energy or stored for future use.

Insulin resistance: A condition in which a person's body tissues have a lowered response to insulin. It is like it has built up tolerance (or "resistance") to the hormone, making it less effective. See Diabetes.

Ischemia: Areas of reduced oxygen supply due to lack of blood supply.

Kidney disease: The gradual loss of kidney function. Failure of the kidneys to filter waste products from the blood properly. When kidney disease impairs the kidney function and lasts longer than three months, this is called Chronic Renal Insufficiency (CRI).

Lipid profile: See *lipoprotein*.

Lipoprotein (LDL & HDL): A group of proteins capable of mixing with water or blood that combine with fat to transport it through your bloodstream. LDL is low-density lipoprotein (sometimes called *bad* cholesterol) and HDL is high-density lipoprotein (sometimes called *good* cholesterol). You want your lipid profile cholesterol report to have "Low LDL, High HDL."

Lipoprotein(a): A type of lipoprotein that helps transport the cholesterol in the blood. What makes this "(a)" one different is that it resembles the *bad* cholesterol (LDL) and other particles that promote clotting. It also promotes inflammation and this is not good to have circulating inside your blood vessels. You should be tested for Lp(a) levels if you have been diagnosed with heart disease but don't have "traditional risk factors" or if you have family history of early heart disease. If your level of Lp(a) is 30 mg/dL or higher, your risk for heart disease is higher.

Lipoprotein lipase: A substance that increases the breakdown of cholesterol. It can lead to the accumulation of fat in the abdominal region.

Menopause: Menopause is diagnosed when a woman has not had a menstrual period for 12 consecutive months. It's associated with lower levels of the hormone estrogen. As women age, especially after menopause, the proportion of body fat in the midsection increases.

Microvasculature: See *coronary arteries*.

Microvascular disease: Due to lack of blood flow to the heart from dysfunction of the microvasculature. It is the main difference between women and men with CAD. See Coronary microvascular dysfunction.

MINOCA: The acronym for: *myocardial infarction with no obstructive coronary artery disease.*

Myocardial infarction: See *heart attack*.

Nervous system: See *autonomic nervous system*.

Nitric oxide: A compound produced by the lining of the interior wall of the arteries. It helps widen the blood vessels.

Oxidation of LDL: An example of oxidation is rusting of metals. You don't want your LDL to get too oxidized because it makes it even more damaging. You can help to combat this by eating more antioxidants like those in colorful fruits and vegetables.

Palpitations: A strong heartbeat or a racing pulse indicating increased blood pressure. It's the sensation that your heart is beating fast or like butterflies on your chest.

Peripheral vascular disease (PVD): A disease of the arteries that supply the rest of your body, beyond your heart. Also known as *peripheral arterial disease* (PAD).

Plaque: Mix of cholesterol, calcium, and scar tissue. (Whenever you see the word atherosclerosis in this book think about plaque.) Plaque formation is stimulated by many things, including smoking. The plaque inside the arteries can be stable or unstable plaques. The less stable the plaque, the more likely it is to break apart or "rupture" and cause a heart attack.

Physical activity (PA): Being active means a lifestyle that includes physical activity equivalent to walking more than three miles per day at 3-4 miles per hour, in addition to the activities of daily living.

Postmenopausal: After the menopause. Menopause is diagnosed with a women has not menstrual period for 12 consecutive months.

Prinzmetal angina: Intermittent spasms of the coronary arteries that causes chest pain.

Processed foods: See *ultra-processed foods.*

Pulmonary congestion: Often referred to as fluid or water in the lungs and can result from diastolic dysfunction ("stiff heart").

Pulse: See *heart rate.*

Remodeling: After a heart attack there is damage to your heart. As part of the healing process, there will be remodeling of the heart that is manifested as changes in size and function of the heart.

Statins: Medications that appear to reduce overall heart disease risk. Statins lower the amount of LDL in the blood by reducing the production of cholesterol in the liver. Some of the statins include atorvastatin (Lipitor), fluvastatin (LEscol), lovastatin (Mevacor), pitavastatin (Livalo), pravastatin (Pravachol) rosuvastatin (Crestor), and simvastatin (Zocor).

Stent: A small metal cylinder that is inserted inside an artery to release a blockage due to plaque.

Stiff heart: See *diastolic dysfunction.*

Stress test: An exercise stress test that is one of the most commonly used tests to reveal hidden problems in the heart making your heart work harder. It is similar to what a mechanic does when checking your car engine. The most common one is the Exercise Treadmill Test (ETT) where you walk or run on a treadmill or pedal on a stationary bike. During this test, your doctor monitors blood pressure, heart rate, and your heart electrical activity for changes that suggest a blockage of blood flow to the heart.

Stroke: A condition that happens when your brain doesn't get enough oxygenated blood.

Tachycardia includes:

- SVT (supraventricular tachycardia): Rapid pulse coming from the upper chambers of your heart (the atria).
- Premature contractions: A premature beat causes your heart to beat early before the next regular heartbeat. They can go unnoticed but some patients experience palpitations, dizziness, and lightheadedness. Some others experience a strong heartbeat and sometimes the sensation that the heart stop beating momentarily.

- Atrial fibrillation: In this type of arrhythmia the heartbeat that originates in the upper chambers of the heart is irregular, unorganized and rapid. This make the upper chambers of the heart quiver instead of beating effectively.
- Atrial flutter: A more organized arrhythmia that originates in the atrium. Although treated similarly to atrial fibrillation, in this condition the heartbeat appears more organized.
- Ventricular tachycardia: Originates in the ventricle. Mostly seen in women with heart disease. The treatment varies and it depends on symptoms and other medical conditions. This is considered a serious rhythm problem that can become a life-threatening problem. This arrhythmia requires immediate attention.

Takotsubo syndrome: Microvascular constriction that reduces blood flow to the heart muscle

Triglycerides (TGs): The most common type of fat in your body. When your blood level of TGs are too high, this is a risk for heart disease.

Ultra-processed foods: Ultra-processed foods include everything that has been milled, canned, cooked, frozen, or dehydrated; however, these on their own do not necessarily make them bad. What makes them bad is the number of changes the ingredients go through as food manufacturers improve flavor, color, and shelf life to make it a harmful processed food. For example, milling of grains will remove the bran and the germ which contain most of the healthy fiber, protein, vitamins, and minerals. Another example is the addition of sugar or salt to food which makes it less healthy. Canned foods, sugar coated dried fruits, soda, sugary or savory packaged snack foods, packaged breads and pastries, breaded chicken nuggets and fish, and instant noodle soups are all examples of ultra-processed foods. Look for other additives and trans fats listed in the Nutrition Facts table (See Appendix I for a table of the most common food additives).

Vasospastic disease: Spasm of the main branches of the coronary arteries.

Ventricles: See *chambers of the heart.*

Visceral adipose tissue: See *adipose tissue.*

> Prevention is the most important intervention.
>
> #PreventTheStent

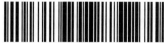
56713461R00087

Made in the USA
Columbia, SC
01 May 2019